VOL. II

DPH, 1975

A Supplement to The Broad Range of Use of Diphenylhydantoin

BIBLIOGRAPHY AND REVIEW

Samuel Bogoch, M.D., Ph.D.
Jack Dreyfus, B.A., LL.D. (Hon.)

The Dreyfus Medical Foundation

The Dreyfus Medical Foundation is a charitable
foundation and has no financial interest in
diphenylhydantoin, either directly or indirectly.

The Two Books

DPH, 1975 is a supplement to The Broad Range of Use of Diphenylhydantoin, and should be read in combination with it. Neither book is complete without the other.

The Broad Range of Use of Diphenylhydantoin, first published in 1970, will be referred to in this book as Vol. I. It covers the period from 1937 to 1970 and is arranged chronologically.

DPH, 1975 is based mainly on studies published in the last five years. In addition to its own Tables of Content, it contains a Combined Clinical Table (for the two volumes) and a combined Subject Index. There are many cross references from DPH, 1975 to Vol. I, but none in the other direction.

The purpose in these books is to bring to the physician much of the published information on the many clinical uses[1] of DPH and its basic mechanisms of action.

[1]Clinical uses other than in epilepsy. The reference library of the Foundation is accessible to interested persons.

In the Appendix

Some matters, sociomedical in nature, are discussed briefly in the Appendix, p. 95. They include the origin of the interest of The Dreyfus Medical Foundation in DPH; cooperation with and from Federal Health Agencies; the fact that DPH's only FDA approved indication is for epilepsy; the use of DPH by physicians throughout the world for a wide range of disorders, and estimates of this use in the United States by independent survey.

DPH, 1975 — *Table of Contents*

Clinical Uses of Diphenylhydantoin

Basic Mechanisms of Action

(continued)

DPH, 1975 AND THE BROAD RANGE OF USE OF DIPHENYLHYDANTOIN

Combined (Clinical) Table of Contents

Background and Distinctive Characteristics of DPH

Background

In its first clinical trials, in epilepsy, diphenylhydantoin was so effective that it was labeled an anticonvulsant, and the concept that it was a single-purpose medicine persisted for many years. However, from the beginning, other uses were being found for DPH.

Starting in 1938, a series of published works indicated that DPH had salutary effects on personality, memory, mood, cooperativeness and emotional stability. As early as 1944, Silverman, in a double-blind study with prisoners, reported that DPH was more effective than any other substance tried, in improving sleep disturbances, sense of well-being and cooperativeness. Other studies found DPH effective in emotions related to fear and anger, and in depression. It was observed that these improvements in thought, mood and behavior were achieved without sedation.

As early as 1940, Shapera found DPH effective in conditions of involuntary movements and in the treatment of migraine. By 1942, Shulman had reported DPH therapeutic in intractable bronchial asthma and, in the same year, Bergouignan observed DPH useful in trigeminal neuralgia. Bodkin, in 1945, reported DPH successful in the treatment of pruritus ani. In 1948, Fabrykant found DPH effective in stabilizing labile diabetes. In 1950, Harris and Kokernot reported that DPH controlled ventricular tachycardias in dogs. The first clinical report of DPH's usefulness in ventricular tachycardias was by Leonard in 1958. In 1961, Isaacs found DPH effective, when other substances had failed, in the treatment of continuous muscle fiber activity. A series of studies have demonstrated that DPH is useful in a variety of painful conditions – from mild headache to such severe conditions as trigeminal neuralgia and thalamic pain.

Today, DPH is no longer thought of as a single-purpose medicine but is broadly known as a stabilizer of bioelectrical activity, or a cell stabilizer. Clinically, it is referred to as a stabilizer or a normalizer.

The recognition of DPH as a multi-purpose medicine has opened new areas for exploration and it is being found useful for an increasingly wide range of disorders. (See Table of Contents and Subject Index.)

Because DPH is useful in so many medical disciplines an over-all summary is impractical.[1] However, a review of some of its distinctive characteristics follows.

[1]Individual summaries will be found in the sections on Thought, Mood and Behavior, Cardiovascular Disorders, Muscle Disorders, Treatment of Pain and Basic Mechanisms of Action.

Distinctive Characteristics

DPH has distinctive characteristics which, taken together, set it apart from other substances.

1. DPH regulates bioelectrical activity at the individual cell level.[1] This action at a level fundamental to all body functions helps explain how DPH achieves its therapeutic effects in a wide range of disorders.

2. DPH is selective in its action in that it corrects inappropriate electrical activity, but does not affect normal function.[1]

3. When cells are overstimulated electrically or chemically a hyperexcitable state develops, referred to as post-tetanic potentiation, which can develop into spontaneous firing, referred to as post-tetanic after-discharge. DPH has a corrective effect on both these conditions.[1] This delineation of a basic action of DPH helps in understanding how repetitive messages of pain are offset or reduced; it may also explain how repetitive and uncontrolled thinking is decreased.

4. DPH has regulatory effects on endocrine and metabolic processes.[2] It has anti-anoxic effects,[3] and it has anti-toxic properties.[4]

5. DPH has been found to be effective in both hyperexcitable and hypoexcitable conditions.[5]

6. In therapeutic doses DPH is not a sedative, nor is it an artificial stimulant.

7. DPH's action is prompt. Taken orally, it is effective within an hour, intravenously within a few minutes.[6]

8. DPH is non-habit forming.

9. DPH's wide range of safety has been established over a thirty-seven year period.

[1]Stabilization of Bioelectrical Activity, p. 57.
[2]Other Regulatory Effects of DPH, p. 77.
[3]Anti-anoxic Effects of DPH, p. 66.
[4]Anti-toxic Effects of DPH, p. 85.
[5]Related basic mechanism studies—Stabilization of Bioelectrical Activity, p. 57, and Preservation of Energy Compounds in Brain, p. 69.
[6]These clinical observations are confirmed by a variety of quantitative measures.

Clinical Uses of Diphenylhydantoin

Thought, Mood
and Behavior Disorders

SUMMARY

The growth of understanding of the therapeutic value of diphenylhydantoin in thought, mood and behavior disorders dates back to the first paper, in 1938, of Merritt and Putnam.[1] The progress in this field from 1938 to 1970 is reviewed in Vol. I, p. 19-28, in which fifty-three studies are arranged chronologically. Here, in Vol. II, recent studies of the last five years are reviewed.

Basic mechanism studies, with the work of the last five years, are consistent with and make easier to understand the clinical observations of the effectiveness of DPH.

The reader will find relevant the section, "Stabilization of Bioelectrical Activity,"[2] in which it is demonstrated that DPH corrects hyperexcitability, as in post-tetanic potentiation or post-tetanic repetitive discharge, in single cells or in groups of cells. This corrective action is achieved without affecting initial appropriate single impulse, or without affecting normal transmission of electrical impulse.

Of further interest is the section, "Preservation of Energy Compounds in Brain,"[3] in which it is shown that DPH preserves ATP, creatine phosphate and glucose. Of additional interest is the section, "Anti-anoxic Effects of DPH,"[4] in which DPH is shown to have a protective effect against oxygen lack; also the section, "Other Regulatory Effects of DPH,"[5] in which it is shown that DPH has a regulatory effect on norepinephrine, acetylcholine, GABA, calcium metabolism, serotonin, insulin, glucagon and blood sugar; and the observations that DPH increases cerebral blood flow.[6]

Clinically, DPH has a calming effect on the overactive brain. Symptoms of this condition are preoccupation, multiple thinking, and flashes and fragments of thoughts coming and going. DPH reduces this uncontrolled activity enabling more normal thinking processes to be restored. This effect is usually achieved within an hour, and without sedation.

Anger and fear and related emotions are usually found in combination with the overactive brain. Emotional states related to anger for which DPH is therapeutic are impatience, impulsiveness, irritability, aggression, hostility, rage and violence. Emotional states related to fear for which DPH is therapeutic are worry, anxiety, guilt, pessimism and depression. Although these excessive anger and fear states are decreased or eliminated by DPH, realistic reactions of anger and fear are not interfered with.

Sleep disturbances found in combination with the overactive brain fall into two general categories. The first and most frequent category is symptomatized by difficulty in falling asleep because of over-thinking, light sleep accompanied by unpleasant dreams and frequent nightmares, and insufficient sleep. A second category is symptomatized by excessive sleep, so-called avoidance sleep. Relief from both types of sleep disturbances is usually prompt with DPH.

DPH is effective with extremes of mood ranging from depression to the hyperexcitable state. These apparent disparate effects are observed in the overactive impatient individual who is calmed by DPH, and the tired energyless individual who has a return to normal energy levels. These clinical effects are supported by basic mechanism studies.[7]

Somatic symptoms associated with thought, mood and behavior disorders are usually relieved by DPH. Among those most frequently observed are headaches, gastrointestinal disorders, pain in back of neck and other pain, shortness of breath, trembling, muscle spasms, skin disorders, and problems with weight. DPH has been found useful in the treatment of acute alcoholism and in the prevention of alcoholism.

[1] Ref. 557, p. 19, Vol. I.

[2] P. 57. Ref. 90, 250, 257, 289, 365, 458, 467, 468, 472, 789, 885, 954, 955, 1197, 1198, 1221, 1291, 1343, 1400, 1467, 1469, 1494, 1580, 1602.

[3] P. 69. Ref. 17, 37, 483, 739, 1071.

[4] P. 66. Ref. 118, 164, 263, 717, 804, 1160, 1216, 1374, 1419, 1576, 1591.

[5] P. 77. Ref. 454, 522, 532, 573, 575, 629, 789, 872, 885, 909, 924, 1015, 1021, 1062, 1092, 1108, 1109, 1131, 1154, 1220, 1222, 1269, 1272, 1273, 1274, 1282, 1327, 1330, 1355, 1404, 1406, 1417, 1454, 1509, 1567, 1608, 1642, 1644.

[6] Ref. 790, 938, 1216, 1560.

[7] See "Stabilization of Bioelectrical Activity," p. 57, and "Preservation of Energy Compounds in Brain," p. 69.

Thought, Mood
and Behavior Disorders

Recent Studies

Work of the last five years includes, in addition to general studies, studies of the effect of DPH on violence and uncontrolled behavior, DPH's effect on concentration and cognitive function in the young and the aged, its effect on patients with hypoglycemia, its effect on cerebral blood flow in the aged, on compulsive eating, on drug withdrawal, and on learning functions in retarded children.

In the first two studies that follow, the effectiveness of DPH is demonstrated by quantitative laboratory methods.

Stambaugh and Tucker use a recently developed technique, the radioimmunoassay method, to demonstrate that DPH regulates plasma insulin levels. In the other study (a basic mechanisms study), Delgado, Mora and Sanguinetti, using radiotelemetry, record the ability of DPH to eliminate post-tetanic repetitive after-discharge in the brain of the awake and functioning rhesus monkey.

Hypoglycemia

STAMBAUGH and TUCKER, *Diabetes* (1974),[1583] describe the successful treatment, with diphenylhydantoin, of five patients with functional hypoglycemia previously unresponsive to dietary management.

Among the symptoms, typical of the hypoglycemic patient, were chronic anxiety, extreme lethargy, chills, frequent nausea, sensory deficits and other neurological complaints. These symptoms disappeared during DPH therapy, along with the hypoglycemia.

Clinical reversal of hypoglycemia was observed in all five cases. In addition, laboratory tests confirmed this observation in both six-hour glucose

tolerance and insulin level tests, performed before and after DPH therapy.

Detailed data presented for all five patients in terms of six-hour plasma glucose tests and plasma insulin values[1] are shown in the figures which follow.

As seen in these figures, DPH demonstrated a regulatory effect on both plasma insulin and plasma glucose in that it brought abnormally high plasma insulin levels down into the normal range and abnormally low plasma glucose levels up into the normal range.

[1]This demonstration of DPH's regulatory effect on plasma insulin and plasma glucose levels supports the work of Fabrykant[91,92,430] and Wilson[382] on the clinical improvement with DPH in labile diabetes. See also Ref. 733, 909, 924, 959, 1015, 1092, 1154, 1193, 1222, 1272, 1274, 1275, 1354, 1355, 1404, 1509.

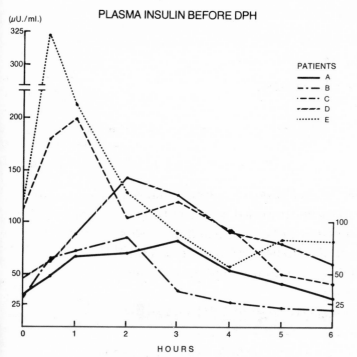

Demonstration of abnormally large insulin response to a glucose load in hypoglycemic patients.

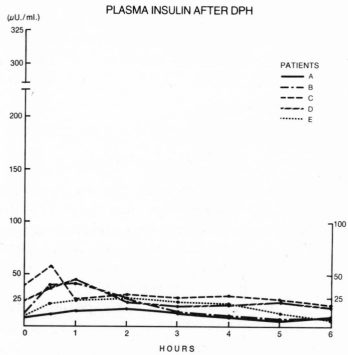

With DPH, the same patients do not have a hyperinsulin response to the glucose load. The response is in the normal range.

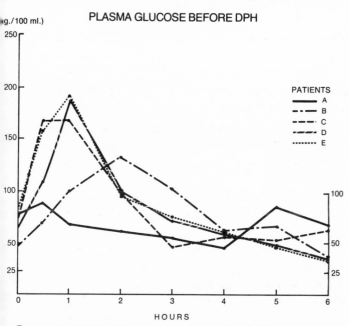

Demonstration that in hypoglycemic patients, blood sugar falls to abnormally low levels in response to a glucose load.

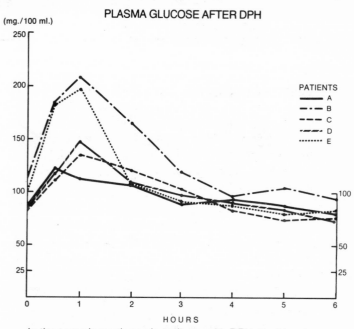

In the same hypoglycemic patients, with DPH, the blood sugar returns to normal levels in response to a glucose load.

REPETITIVE AFTER-DISCHARGE
(basic mechanisms study)

DELGADO, MORA and SANGUINETTI, *Personal Communication* (1973), [954] studied the effect of DPH on after-discharge in the amygdala of the brain of awake active rhesus monkeys.

Earlier work[953] had shown that certain forms of abnormal spread of electrical after-discharge could be induced in the monkey by intracerebral electrical stimulation in several areas of the brain,

including the thalamus and amygdala. Electrical after-discharge was decreased dramatically in the thalamus by DPH. The strong effect of DPH upon limiting the spread of electrical after-discharge in the cerebral cortex was also noted.

In the present study, with repeated electrical stimulation sufficiently close together, in this case ten minutes apart, repetitive after-discharge could be obtained with 100% reliability. These after-discharges are analogous to the post-tetanic potentiation and post-tetanic after-discharges described in the studies of others. Certain abnormal behavioral

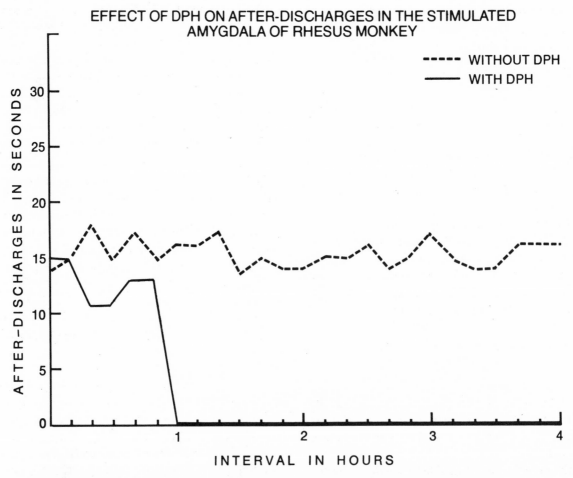

EFFECT OF DPH ON AFTER-DISCHARGES IN THE STIMULATED AMYGDALA OF RHESUS MONKEY

- - - - WITHOUT DPH
——— WITH DPH

Demonstration of the ability of DPH to eliminate post-tetanic after-discharge, within one hour, in an alert and functioning rhesus monkey.

sequences accompanied the measurable after-discharges from the amygdala.

Intramuscular or intracerebral injection of DPH was found to completely prevent these electrical after-discharges. (See accompanying Figure.)

The time course of action of DPH in these experiments is of interest. DPH showed some effect in reducing after-discharge fifteen to thirty minutes after injection, and produced complete abolition of after-discharges by one hour after injection.

The authors note that in all animals, no changes were recorded in the normal spontaneous electrical activity when DPH was given. However, when the abnormal state of after-discharge was induced, DPH was found to prevent this after-discharge.[1]

[1]This study demonstrates, in an awake and functioning animal, the corrective action of DPH on hyperexcitability. The time course of this effect, correction within one hour, is consistent with therapeutic effects seen in man.

GENERAL

ALVAREZ, in a book titled *"Nerves in Collision"* (1972),[761] reviews his twenty-five years of experience in the use of diphenylhydantoin for a wide variety of disorders.

In this book, the author reports on the successful use of DPH in the treatment of abdominal pain, alcoholism, anorexia nervosa, anxiety, bed wetting, belching (violent), blackouts, confusion, depression, dizzy spells, fatigue (extreme), fear, fever, head pain, involuntary movements, migraine-like headaches, nightmares, nervousness, premature ejaculation, rage, tension and violent outbursts.

TURNER, *Drugs and Cerebral Function* (1970),[1626] in reporting on the effects of diphenylhydantoin on emotionally disturbed children, states that those of us who prescribe DPH have become so accustomed to finding marked improvement in these children that we almost take it for granted that everyone knows of these effects and prescribes the DPH accordingly.

Typical of the problems of these children are hostility, destructiveness, hyperkinesis, inability to get along with others and poor school adjustments. In a recent group of nine emotionally disturbed children, the author reports that treatment with DPH resulted in improvements in seven cases ranging from substantial to complete elimination of symptoms. In one case there was a substantial temporary improvement, and in one case no effect was observed.

BOZZA, in a detailed paper presented at the *Fourth Italian National Congress of Child Neuropsychiatry* (1971),[863] reports on an individual basis on twenty-one brain damaged retarded children who were observed for periods of from twelve to thirty-six months. In a majority of the cases DPH was tried. The author concluded that DPH and vitamins materially improved the expected intellectual growth rate of these retarded children. (See also Ref. 8, 355, 373 and 1626.)

JONAS, *American Journal of Psychiatry* (1969),[1189] who had reported on twelve years of experience with the use of diphenylhydantoin in his book "Ictal and Subictal Neurosis," comments in a letter to the editor of the American Journal of Psychiatry that every investigator who has prescribed DPH over a period of time has found remarkable reversal of symptoms on occasion ranging from the complete disappearance of anxiety to structural changes in the character makeup of the patient.

LOOKER and CONNERS, *Archives of General Psychiatry* (1970),[1304] report on three children in whom diphenylhydantoin was effective to a marked degree in the treatment of severe temper tantrums. In each case the response to DPH was prompt. The children had been previously treated with dextroamphetamine sulfate, to which none of them had any beneficial response.

The children, a seven-year-old girl, a nine-year-old boy and a twelve-year-old girl, were followed-up six months later and the marked improvement had persisted. In two of the cases, when the parents had forgotten to give DPH, deterioration was noted within twenty-four to forty-eight hours. This deterioration was promptly corrected with the reinstitution of DPH.

The authors then conducted a double-blind study with placebo on seventeen subjects, ranging in age from five-and-a-half to fourteen years, who had periodic episodes of misbehavior characterized by temper tantrums, fire-setting, cruelty to animals, homicidal assaultiveness, stealing and bizarre fugue-like states.

Premeasures.—Initial screening measures included the WISC, the Lincoln-Oseretsky Test of Motor Development, the Goodenough Draw-A-Man Test and the Bender Gestalt Test. Parent and teacher symptom checklists were used for initial screening. The Hollingshead Social Index Scale was used. A series of neurological examinations were given. *Postmeasures.*—Subjects were examined with Porteus Maze Tests, Continuous Performance Tests, and parent and school questionnaires. Visual evoked potentials were also obtained.

It was the impression of the authors that among the patients "there were *some* who responded rather dramatically, as in the case histories presented earlier." However, "no statistically significant group changes were attributable to drug effect." This led the authors to conclude that further work was needed to distinguish those types which would respond to DPH. (Also see Conners, et al.)[913]

STEPHENS and SHAFFER, *The Journal of Clinical Pharmacology* (1973). [1592] In an earlier paper[700] the authors had reported on the successful treatment with diphenylhydantoin of thirty private psychiatric outpatients. This study had been done on a double-blind basis and there had been significantly favorable response in symptoms such as anxiety, irritability, impatience and explosive temper.

About two years later, ten of this group of patients agreed to participate in a double-blind study of DPH for four consecutive two-week periods. Two doses were used, 100 mg t.i.d. and 5 mg t.i.d., the latter dose serving essentially as a placebo. Half of the ten patients were started on DPH, 5 mg t.i.d., for the first two-week period, and the other half with 100 mg t.i.d. for the first two-week period. Thereafter for the eight-weeks study they were alternated on these two doses.

Consistent with the previous study, 100 mg t.i.d. of DPH proved significantly more effective than the placebo dosage in relieving symptoms of anxiety, anger and irritability as assessed both by self-ratings and physicians' ratings of change.

DANIEL, *Geriatrics* (1970),[938] states that symptoms of confusion which are so common in the aged often are caused by underlying physical illness, frequently cardiac and respiratory disorders resulting in cerebral anoxia. He states that diphenylhydantoin is therapeutically useful in this group, yet it is often overlooked.[1]

Among the symptoms of confusion so common in the aged are: 1) disorientation, often not of person but in particular of time, place and space; 2) lack of attention and concentration; 3) fluctuation in state of consciousness; 4) memory loss, particulary of current events; 5) poor performance when tested on immediate retention and recall; and 6) impairment of conventional judgment.

The author states that although problems of insufficient cerebral blood flow are well known in the aged, direct measurement of cerebral blood flow is at best difficult.[2] However, the author states that symptoms of insufficient cerebral blood flow are identifiable clinically. Among these symptoms are irritability, restlessness, mental confusion and sometimes severe depression. The author notes that after cerebrovascular accident the patient often has paresthesias and tingling. He states that DPH not only frequently gives relief from the paresthesias, but that mental symptoms also improve.

The author states experience has shown that the improving mental state of the patient on DPH is a reasonable guide to over-all improvement in cerebral function.[3]

[1]Occasionally a study is directly relevant in two separate clinical areas. This study also appears under Cardiovascular Disorders.

[2]For other work on the effect of DPH in Cerebral Blood Flow, see Ref. 790, 1216, 1560.

[3]This discussion of DPH by Daniel is part of a larger study of other substances entitled, "Psychiatric drug use and abuse in the aged."

VIOLENT BEHAVIOR

MALETSKY, *Medical Times* (1972), [1329] states that it is currently fashionable to ascribe the roots of violence to social ills. The role of brain dysfunction has been relatively neglected until recently.

The author reports on a study of twenty-two patients with the syndrome referred to as episodic dyscontrol. In describing this syndrome he states that the subjects usually have a history of hyperactivity and poor school performance as children, aggression towards other children and animals and firesetting. Truancy and petty stealing frequently lead them to grand larceny, assault and battery and even murder. Other typical symptoms are traffic violations and recklessness. The author states that central to this dyscontrol syndrome is the "storm of violence." Upon minimal or even no provocation these patients lose control, wrecking property and directing violence against anyone in their way. These "storms" are directed against close members of the family as well as society. Frequently following such "storms of violence" these persons have extreme feelings of remorse.

Twenty-two patients with episodic dyscontrol were treated with diphenylhydantoin. Tabulation of the results of this treatment was based on the author's observations and, in addition, was based on reports of relatives and friends of the patient. It seemed implausible to the author that a bias would exist in these reports since the patients had all been through futile drug trials in the past.

The results with DPH were so good that the author calls attention to the fact that this was not a "controlled" study. (Later these effects were confirmed in a controlled study. See below.)

The tabulation of results indicated that nineteen of twenty-two subjects, or 86%, achieved a result equal to or better than "good response." Fifteen of these achieved an excellent response with virtually complete absence of attacks. This response usually occurred within the first two weeks and persisted thereafter. Data collected at twelve months showed that all cases responding to DPH remained free of violent outbreaks.

The author finds it interesting to note that none of the patients claimed to have lost the ability to *feel* anger, but that they were better able to prevent its escalation.

MALETSKY and KLOTTER, *Diseases of the Nervous System* (1974), [1328] in a controlled study, found diphenylhydantoin significantly effective (p less than .01) in twenty-two patients with episodic dyscontrol syndrome.

The authors state that this study, with placebo, confirms the earlier work of Maletsky in which he found DPH highly effective in the treatment of this syndrome. As a result of these studies, the authors conclude that DPH should be tried in patients with episodic dyscontrol syndrome.

DIAMOND and YARYURA-TOBIAS, *Paper presented at the Fifth World Congress of Psychiatry* (1971),[961] found diphenylhydantoin effective in the treatment of violent and aggressive behavior in schizophrenics without epilepsy. Twenty-two patients were studied.

The authors state that DPH has been reported to be therapeutic not only for epilepsy but for disorders of the central and peripheral nervous system, cardiac arrhythmias, diabetes, arterial hypertension, asthma and some skin diseases. They state that from the neuropsychiatric viewpoint it is interesting to know that DPH exerts a regularizing effect on human behavior, irritability and anxiety and that it also has an antidepressant action. Aggressive attitude and violent behavior have also been improved by DPH.

The authors state that as early as 1943, Kalinowsky and Putnam[186] observed an improvement of the excitability and excitation of psychotic patients. Some benefits were seen by Freyhan[110] in 1945, by Kubanek and Rowell[201] in 1946 and by Haward[697] in 1969 and negative results were reported by Klein and Greenberg[196] in 1967.

The purpose of the present investigation was to study the action of DPH on psychotics without epilepsy who had symptoms of violent, impulsive, destructive and aggressive behavior. Patients with severe depression and obsessive-compulsive personalities were also included in the study. Some of the patients had EEG disturbances but they were not epileptics and nine of the patients had functional hypoglycemia curves.

With DPH, in doses up to 300 mg a day, violent behavior was well controlled in all cases of schizophrenia, eleven with excellent results and seven with moderate results. A slight improvement in their depression was noticed in five schizophrenic patients. In the cases with neurotic depression and obsessive-compulsive neurosis, the results were negative. The beneficial effects of DPH were observed not only by the investigator and patient, but also by the patient's family.

The authors state that it is necessary to underline that all therapeutic methods used by the patients prior to DPH administration were ineffective. DPH was the variable that changed their behavioral symptoms.

BACH-Y-RITA, LION, CLIMENT and ERVIN, *American Journal of Psychiatry* (1971),[787] reported that in the course of two years they had seen 130 patients with a wide range of complaints pertaining to assaultive and destructive acts. Diphenylhydantoin was found useful whether or not EEG ab-

normalities were displayed by the patients. Phenothiazines were also found useful. As a result, many patients were maintained on a regimen of DPH and phenothiazines for long periods. Psychotherapy, group or individual, was also found useful.

SOLOMON and KLEEMAN, *California Medicine* (1971),[1569] in reporting seven cases of episodic dyscontrol syndrome, comment separately on the only two in which diphenylhydantoin was given. In both cases the patient's behavior was markedly improved.

In the case detailed, a 39-year-old woman entered the hospital because of repeated attacks of wild uncontrolled behavior. Without warning, she would be assailed by intense feelings of either rage or sexual excitement. In rage, she usually attacked her husband. In sexual excitement, she sought partners wherever she could find them and her demands were insatiable. Prolonged psychotherapy and tranquilizing medication had proved ineffective. DPH caused a remarkable improvement in this patient's behavior and she returned to reasonable conduct.

PINTO, SIMOPOULOS, McGEE, UHLENHUTH and DEROSA (1974),[1415] in a study of thirty-two severely regressed chronic schizophrenic patients, found that diphenylhydantoin in doses of 250-350 mg per day, when added to phenothiazine, was more effective than the phenothiazine by itself in reducing irritability, aggression and negative behavior. (See also Simopoulos, Pinto, Uhlenhuth, McGee and DeRosa.)[1551]

COGNITIVE FUNCTION

HAWARD, *Drugs and Cerebral Function* (1970),[1139] studied the effect of diphenylhydantoin upon performance in a complex task, subject to fatigue, in twelve college students who had concentration difficulties. A double-blind crossover procedure was followed. The students were given a task in which each subject received two hours of training in an air traffic control simulator. On two subsequent two-hour trials, each subject received either 150 mg of DPH or placebo.

DPH was found to be significantly effective in delaying the onset of fatigue and accompanying errors. The author notes that although many substances have been used to improve concentration over the past pentade, these substances are usually stimulants. Although DPH improved concentration significantly, it produced none of the effects of a stimulant.

The author notes that these findings are in accord with the observations of Dreyfus[707] that poor concentration can result from forced ruminative thinking, or the "turned-on mind," and that this can be corrected by DPH.

SMITH and LOWREY, *Drugs, Development and Cerebral Function* (1972),[1564] suggest that improvement in cognitive performance can be due to improved ability to concentrate. Using standard IQ tests to measure ability to perform the authors compared the effects of diphenylhydantoin and placebo on twenty general hospital employee volunteers with no evidence of CNS disorders.

The test was done on a double-blind crossover basis against placebo, and two retests were made. DPH, 100 mg three times daily, improved Verbal Scale and Full Scale scores at highly significant levels (.0005) and the Performance Scale improvement was significant (.01). The authors suggest that the validity of this latter result should be tempered by the possibility of the influence of practice effects.

The authors note that although they used an entirely different method, their findings are consistent with those obtained by Haward[1139] by means of perceptual and vigilance tests.

HAWARD, *Revue de Medicine Aeronautique et Spatiale* (1973),[1140] found that diphenylhydantoin

significantly improved the performance of three separate groups of pilots in simulated flying and radar target-fixing tasks.

The author introduces the subject by saying that previous experiments[585,1139] have shown that single doses of DPH are able to counteract the onset of mental fatigue in an Air Traffic Control task. Smith and Lowrey[1564] have also shown that DPH can improve performance on IQ tests. These findings suggest that DPH may also have some value in pilots suffering from operational fatigue, or other conditions in which intellectual processes or work performance is temporarily impaired.

The author states that one of the major difficulties in tasks of vigilance, attention or concentration is to demonstrate impairment within a practical period of time. This is because, in conditions of apparent maximum concentration, the operator still retains a reserve of uncommitted neurons. These enable him to compensate, in the early stages at least, for the effects of fatigue, etc. Therefore, in order to demonstrate the onset of this decrement of mental skills, it is necessary to load the operator to the limit of his channel capacity.

In the present study three groups of pilots were included, twenty-two commercial pilots, eighteen military pilots and nineteen private pilots. Two absorbing tasks were required of the pilots in an attempt to reach full channel capacity. The first was a standard flight simulation procedure. The second task consisted of monitoring and responding to a new type of forward-looking radar.

The pilots were scored on their ability to bring the simulated aircraft position to correctly intercept a moving target. The time of performing the task as well as the number of correct responses were measured. Sixty minutes before each task 150 mg of DPH was given.

With DPH the test results showed significant improvement in performance both in terms of lessened time spent and the increased number of correct responses made when compared to the tests without DPH. In all three groups the improvement was significant.

The author states that he chose DPH for this test not only because of its already established efficacy in improving cognitive processes, but because other substances which have been tried for this purpose, such as amphetamine, pemoline and prolintane, have undesirable side or after effects. In the dosage used for this purpose, DPH has proved to be free of any side reactions. In an earlier paper Haward[1139] mentioned that, "Unlike other substances DPH has a stabilizing effect on the nervous system, acting neither as a stimulant nor as a depressant, but as what has been called a normalizer."

The author concludes that DPH may have a useful role in the maintaining of efficiency of critical aircraft personnel.

SMITH and LOWREY, *Journal of the American Geriatrics Society* (1975),[1565] observed the beneficial effect of diphenylhydantoin upon cognitive function in a group of elderly normal subjects.

The authors note that a growing amount of evidence has accumulated over the past decade demonstrating the beneficial use of DPH on a variety of physical conditions. They also note that several studies have appeared in the last few years which demonstrate that DPH not only assists concentration when impairment in cognitive function is caused by irrelevant ruminative preoccupation, but that it also improves concentration when efficiency is impaired by fatigue.

The authors state that the purpose of the present study was to examine the effect of DPH upon ability to concentrate in a group of elderly people. Standard intelligence tests were used to compare the subjects' abilities to perform with and without DPH. Intelligence improvement was not expected, but it was thought that improved ability to concentrate would show up in better scores on the intelligence tests.

In the present study ten volunteers, four male and six female, average age 69 years, were studied in a double-blind crossover test with placebo control. This crossover design was used to eliminate possible practice effects on performance.

With DPH significant improvement in scores occurred in information, comprehension, digit symbol and full scale IQ. The authors conclude that these significant improvements illustrate the effectiveness of DPH in improving generalized mental functions.

The authors point out that significant similarities exist between their two studies of DPH. In the present study, since only ten subjects were used, the authors suggest that more work be done, particularly since problems with memory are common in the elderly.

The authors note that in addition to Haward's findings, these observations are consistent with the findings of the beneficial effects of DPH on the "turned-on mind" (Worcester County Jail double-blind study, Resnick and Dreyfus).[704]

OTHER DISORDERS

COMPULSIVE EATING

GREEN and RAU, *American Journal of Psychiatry* (1974),[1097] found diphenylhydantoin highly effective in treating ten patients who had three distinct types of symptoms of compulsive eating.

One group was extremely underweight. Sometimes they ate nothing, yet they constantly thought about food. Frequently they would overeat and then would overcorrect this condition by forcing themselves to vomit. Thus they stayed underweight. These patients were considered by the author to come under the category of primary anorexia nervosa.

The second group consisted of persons of normal weight. They were also preoccupied with food and they had a compulsive wish to eat. Their entire lives were structured to avoid exposure to food through various and complicated maneuvers. They occasionally went on eating binges that lasted for hours or days. They would then diet back to normal, unlike group one, who always dieted back to below normal.

Group three consisted of patients who gave in to their strong compulsion to eat. They became overweight over a period of years, some rapidly, some slowly. They were from 150 to 250 pounds above normal weight.

Of the ten patients, nine had abnormal EEGs but none was epileptic. DPH was highly effective in nine of these patients, including the one with normal EEG. The authors give particulars of the successful use of DPH in three remarkable cases, one from each of the groups mentioned. It is apparent that compulsive eating is one of a group of undesirable symptoms, and improvement with DPH in the compulsive eating syndrome coincided with improvement in other symptoms, including depression. In two of the three cases DPH was withdrawn and symptoms returned. When DPH was reinstated, the symptoms disappeared.

LSD FLASHBACKS

THURLOW and GIRVIN, *Canadian Medical Association Journal* (1971),[1616] reported the successful treatment with diphenylhydantoin of two cases of flashbacks (recurrent visual hallucinations after LSD). In one of the cases DPH was given intravenously, and it terminated the flashback while in progress. In the other case DPH was used orally, and within forty-eight hours marked improvement was noted.

In one of the cases the patient had been suffering from flashbacks five months after the discontinuance of all hallucinogenic drugs. She was given chlorpromazine, 25 mg t.i.d., with moderate diminution in the intensity, frequency and affective component of her flashbacks. Big hallucinations continued to occur, but were less terrifying. Chlorpromazine was discontinued and the previous level of flashbacks returned within twenty-four hours.

Two days after discontinuance of chlorpromazine, DPH was instituted, 100 mg t.i.d. The patient was not informed of the nature of the medicine or of its possible effects. Within forty-eight hours she noted a very marked reduction in all types of flashbacks, a complete disappearance of big ones and a reduction of the little ones to a barely discernible level. DPH was discontinued after four months and the patient was followed for eight months with no return of flashback symptoms.

In the other case 100 mg of DPH intravenously terminated a flashback while in progress. Before injecting DPH, saline solution was injected, as a control, with no effect.

ADDICTION

FISHER and DiMINO, *Personal Communication* (1972),[1033] in discussing their clinical experience, report that they found diphenylhydantoin to be useful in their over-all therapeutic approach to withdrawal from addictive agents, including heroin, amphetamines, and alcohol.[1]

[1]See Fertziger, et al.[1026, 1027] on counteraction by DPH of morphine effects in animals.

GILLES DE LA TOURETTE

BARSKY, *Journal of Pediatrics* (1967),[796] reports on the unusual symptom complex known as "Tic Convulsif de Gilles de la Tourette." The author states that the hallmarks of this disorder are involuntary movements beginning in childhood in association with a phenomenon referred to as coprolalia (an irresistible use of obscene language).

In this case of a nine-year-old girl, the parents had observed during the preceding year an alarming increase in sudden, purposeless jerking movements of her body. These would vary from sharp, repetitive head jerks, to arm flexions, eye blinking, or leg kicking. Lately, coprolalia had manifested itself. The child would repeat the same obscene statement over and over again and, although aware of it, could not stop repeating it.

Although otherwise quite normal, the girl's involuntary movements and coprolalia were becoming intolerable and kept her from school. At the time of admission to the hospital the girl appeared to be alert, pleasant and was above average in intelligence. However, she could not sit or stand quietly but was involved in some muscular gyration of arm, leg, face or neck constantly. X-rays of the skull and electroencephalogram did not reveal any significant abnormality. Upon the recommendation of a colleague, Dr. Donald Besant, the patient was treated with diphenylhydantoin, 100 mg t.i.d.

The author states that with DPH there was remarkable improvement within six weeks, and the patient was free of manifestations within six months. DPH was administered for a total of twenty-four months. In a follow-up four years after the discontinuation of DPH, the patient was entirely symptom free.

The author notes that although there are not many cases of this disorder reported in the literature (forty-four cases by Kelman in 1965), his colleagues have not found it uncommon.

Cardiovascular Disorders

SUMMARY

The first evidence that diphenylhydantoin would be useful in cardiology was presented by Harris and Kokernot in 1950 when they showed that it reversed cardiac arrhythmias in dogs. The first evidence that DPH was useful in the treatment of cardiac arrhythmias, in man, was presented in a remarkable paper by Leonard in 1958. These studies, and subsequent studies, of the treatment of cardiac arrhythmias are summarized in Vol. I. They show the progression of use of DPH as a therapeutic substance for cardiac arrhythmias.

Studies that have been published in the last few years greatly increase the understanding of DPH and point to broader uses in cardiovascular disorders. It has been demonstrated that DPH offsets the toxic effects of digitalis without impairing its inotropic benefits. A recent study suggests that DPH may enhance these inotropic benefits.[1] DPH's ability to offset toxic effects of digitalis enables larger amounts of digitalis to be given before toxic levels are reached.

The use of DPH in conduction defects has been further studied.[2] The preponderance of evidence suggests that DPH does not impair conduction. Recent studies indicate that it may improve conduction.[3]

A group of studies in animals indicates that DPH is useful against hypoxia. One of these studies shows that it protects the Purkinje fibers of the heart against oxygen lack. There is evidence that DPH improves coronary blood flow in animals, and there are indications that DPH increases cerebral blood flow in animals and also in man. One study suggests that DPH is useful in the treatment of hypertension in man and another reports that in animals it decreases cardiac calcification.

Consistent throughout both clinical and basic mechanisms studies is the evidence that DPH is rapidly effective, and that it has a wide margin of safety in comparison with other substances.

In addition to its specific actions, DPH has three general properties relevant to the treatment of cardiovascular disorders. These properties are its effectiveness against hypoxia,[4] its effectiveness against pain of a variety of conditions (without impairment of cognitive and motor functions),[5] and its effectiveness against fear and tension.[6]

[1] Ref. 1085.

[2] Ref. 753, 764, 793, 816, 826, 830, 831, 832, 833, 884, 923, 935, 1114, 1120, 1264, 1339, 1390, 1434, 1450, 1488, 1562, 1590, 1645, 1710.

[3] Ref. 753, 764, 793, 816, 826, 830, 831, 884, 935, 1264, 1434, 1488, 1562, 1645, 1710.

[4] Ref. 164, 699, 717, 804, 1160, 1216, 1373, 1576, 1591.

[5] Ref. 3, 9, 14, 15, 16, 31, 40, 48, 54, 66, 68, 78, 81, 111, 112, 113, 114, 129, 160, 161, 175, 180, 202, 214, 224, 227, 235, 304, 315, 317, 329, 330, 338, 380, 384, 386, 420, 422, 429, 465, 518, 543, 551, 564, 583, 586, 587, 605, 611, 633, 693, 707, 727, 732, 744, 747, 748, 881, 883, 1066, 1116, 1171, 1192, 1242, 1243, 1299, 1342, 1360, 1369, 1444, 1501, 1541, 1611, 1657, 1658, 1676.

[6] See Thought, Mood and Behavior, p. 19, Vol. I and p. 8, Vol. II.

CARDIAC ARRHYTHMIAS

Cardiac arrhythmias have been reviewed in Vol. I (pp. 37-45). Many reviews on this subject have been published recently (see below).[1]

In addition to recent studies of the use of DPH in cardiac arrhythmias, there are included herein recent studies showing the effect of DPH in cardiac conduction, myocardial infarction, angina pectoris, hypokalemia, cardioversion, hypertension and cerebral blood flow.

[1] ITALY: Lotto, et al., *Cardiologia Pratica* (1971),[1307] Porciello and Zanini, *Fracastoro* (1971),[1425] Porciello, et al., *Giornale Italiano Cardiologia* (1972).[1426]

SWITZERLAND: Bender, *Schweizerische Medizinische Wochenschrift* (1973),[817] Burckhardt and Sefidpar *Schweizerische Rundschau Medizinische* (1971),[880] Vaughan Williams, *Schweizerische Medizinische Wochenschrift* (1973).[1946]

NETHERLANDS: Van Dijk, *Folia Medica Neerlandica* (1971).[1638]

GERMANY: Herbinger, *Wiener Medizinische Wochenschrift* (1971).[1148]

ROMANIA: Fica, et al., *Medicina Interna* (1971).[1029]

UNITED STATES: American Medical Association on Drugs, *AMA* (1971),[762] Damato, *Progress in Cardiovascular Diseases* (1969),[936] Danzig, *Nebraska Medical Journal* (1971),[941] Doherty, *Annals of Internal Medicine* (1973),[969] Dreifus, *Cardiovascular Therapy, The Art and The Science* (1971),[975] Dreifus and Watanabe, *American Heart Journal* (1970),[972] Dreifus, et al., *American Heart Journal* (1974),[973] Gettes, *American Journal of Cardiology* (1971),[1067] Goldstein, *American Journal of Pharmacy* (1973),[1084] Huffman and Azarnoff, *Rational Drug Therapy* (1974),[1170] Lawrence, *Topics on Medicinal Chemistry* (1970),[1261] Levitt, et al., *Mt. Sinai Journal of Medicine* (1970),[1277] Lown, et al., *Circulation* (1973),[1311] Lucchesi, *University of Michigan Medical Center Journal* (1971),[1312] Mason, et al., *Drugs, Part I and Part II* (1973),[1336] and [1537] Mason, et al., *The Acute Cardiac Emergency-Diagnosis and Management* (1972),[1335] Mason, et al., *Cardiovascular Therapy, The Art and The Science* (1971),[1338] Moss and Patton, *Antiarrhythmic Agents* (1973),[1372] Preston, et al., *Geriatrics* (1973),[1429] Schick and Scheuer, *American Heart Journal* (1974),[1508] Schwender, *Annual Reports in Medicinal Chemistry* (1970),[1515] Smith, *New England Journal of Medicine* (1973).[1563]

ARRHYTHMIAS—DIGITALIS

HANSEN and WAGENER, *Deutsche Medizinische Wochenschrift* (1971),[1121] in a controlled study of 200 patients with DPH and 300 patients without DPH, evaluated the effect of diphenylhydantoin when added to cardiac glycoside administration.

By combining DPH and glycosides, the incidence of arrhythmias was reduced from 21% in the non-DPH group to 2.5% in the DPH-treated group. This significantly enhanced the possibility of achieving adequate digitalization.

The authors state that this clinical experience indicates that DPH administration reduces the toxic effect of glycosides in man without adverse influence on their positive inotropic effect. Thus, the use of DPH improves the chance of effective treatment in heart failure.

GATTENLOHNER and SCHNEIDER, *Munchener Medizinische Wochenschrift* (1969),[1052] reported on the results of their study of cardiac hemodynamics during the intravenous use of diphenylhydantoin. They found that DPH has very good antiarrhythmic efficiency, especially in digitalis-induced arrhythmias where it may be life saving.

The authors state that DPH in the doses which they used (125 and 250 mg per patient) did not change cardiac output or stroke volume.

CHUNG, *Modern Treatment* (1971),[905] in a review of digitalis therapy, states that various clinical investigations have demonstrated that diphenylhydantoin is effective in treating digitalis-induced arrhythmias, including paroxysmal atrial tachycardia, A-V nodal (junctional) rhythm, wandering atrial pacemaker, ventricular bigeminy and multifocal ventricular tachycardia. Most patients respond within three seconds to five minutes with intravenous administration of DPH. The duration of response varies from five minutes to six hours. In-

itial intravenous doses range between 125 and 250 mg for one to three minutes, with electrocardiographic monitoring. When necessary, this same dose may be repeated every five to ten minutes until the desired effect is achieved. After conversion to sinus rhythm or the disappearance of the arrhythmia, oral maintenance doses between 300 and 400 mg daily, in divided doses, are sufficient.

The author states that DPH has prophylactic value when given before direct-current shock to the digitalized patient, since DPH is capable of preventing arrhythmias induced by cardioversion. The author states that DPH is probably the safest and most effective drug in the treatment of all types of digitalis-induced tachyarrhythmias.

STAZI and MARASA, *Annali di Medicina Navale* (1972),[1590] in a review, state that during the past few years diphenylhydantoin has become the drug of choice for use against cardiac arrhythmias due to intoxication from digitalis. The authors state that DPH has the following properties: 1) it suppresses atrial and ventricular hyperexcitability; 2) it reduces increased ventricular automatism; 3) at the usual therapeutic dosage (5 mg/kg), it has little effect on the automatism of the sinus and on intraventricular conduction; 4) it facilitates or leaves unaltered A-V conduction; and 5) it shortens the refractory period.

In addition to its therapeutic action, the authors state that DPH also exerts prophylactic effect. Its preventive administration has been shown to permit up to a 224% increase in the usable dose of digitalis, without interfering with its inotropic benefit.

SMITH and HABER, *New England Journal of Medicine* (1973),[1562] in a review of digitalis toxicity, say that toxic manifestations of digitalis persist as one of the most prevalent adverse drug reactions encountered in clinical practice.

In discussing substances therapeutic in digitalis toxic ectopic arrhythmias, the authors state that diphenylhydantoin is a highly useful drug. It has little adverse effect on sinoatrial rate, atrial conduction, atrioventricular conduction or conduction in the His-Purkinje system. Indeed, DPH may improve sinoatrial block and atrioventricular conduction under some circumstances.

RUMACK, WOLFE and GILFRICH, *British Heart Journal* (1974),[1488] detailed the effective treatment with diphenylhydantoin in a seventeen-year-old patient who attempted suicide with a massive digoxin overdose. Fifty tablets of digoxin (0.25 mg) were ingested.[1] Serum digoxin levels reached 35 ng/ml. Pronounced hyperkalemia[2] was noted fourteen hours after ingestion.

The authors state that though several papers suggest that very large doses of DPH are necessary to overcome digitalis intoxication, they did not find this to be the case. The patient responded to seven doses of 25 mg intravenous DPH over a period of thirty-six hours. Repeated doses of DPH are known to improve A-V conduction, resulting in greater atrial input to the ventricle. The patient had complete heart block early in her course and DPH restored this to a first-degree block.

The authors state that this case and a few others reported indicate that potassium should not be the initial drug of choice as has been suggested in standard toxicology textbooks. They note that low doses of DPH were effective in this case and they suggest that it should be used early in the treatment of acute digoxin overdose.

[1]Seventeen 400 mg tablets of meprobamate had also been ingested.

[2]For a report of beneficial effects of DPH in hypokalemia, see O'Reilly and MacDonald.[1390]

ADAMSKA-DYNIEWSKA, *Polish Medical Journal* (1970),[753] reported on forty-nine patients with chronic heart failure who received diphenylhydantoin (100-300 mg orally) together with cardiac glycosides (deslanoside 0.4 mg or ouabain 0.25 mg, intravenously).

The author states that DPH leveled the digitalis-induced elongation of the atrioventricular conduction and reduced the negative chronotropic action of ouabain, but did not impair the digitalis-improved dynamics of the complete left ventricular systole, as measured by the Q-11A index.

In patients with chronic heart failure, the author states that combined administration of the average clinical doses of cardiac glycosides plus DPH can be applied in clinical conditions which require counteracting of the chrono- and dromotropic action of digitalis, but without any interference with its beneficial effect on heart muscle contractility.

REVIEWS (DIGITALIS)

Levitt, Raines, Sohn, Standaert and Hirshfeld,[1277] Ellis and Dimond,[1007] Smith,[1563] Schwender,[1515] Doherty,[969] Burckhardt and Sefidpar,[880] Schick and Scheuer,[1508] Goldstein,[1084] Huffman and Azarnoff,[1170] and Danzig.[941]

ARRHYTHMIAS—Other

REIMANN, LEMMEL and THEISEN, *Munchener Medizinische Wochenschrift* (1971),[1450] found that in forty-seven of fifty patients diphenylhydantoin eliminated extrasystoles and tachycardias of both atrial and ventricular origin. They noted that A-V conduction was not delayed.

Intravenous injection of 125 to 375 mg was usually immediately effective.

EDDY and SINGH, *British Medical Journal* (1969),[987] treated thirty-seven patients with cardiac arrhythmias with intravenous diphenylhydantoin. Twenty-one had acute myocardial infarctions and sixteen had other conditions. There was a favorable response in eighteen of the twenty-one cases of myocardial infarction and in six of the other sixteen cases.

The authors make note that in a child with Ebstein's anomaly and recurrent supraventricular tachycardia the response to oral DPH was very satisfactory, and when the drug was given for a long period as a prophylactic measure it led to significant improvement.

LESBRE, CATHALA, SALVADOR, FLORIO, LESCURE and MERIEL, *Archives des Maladies du Coeur et des Vaisseaux* (1969),[1264] investigated the antiarrhythmic value of diphenylhydantoin, both clinically and experimentally.

In the clinical study, a variety of arrhythmia disturbances were treated with DPH with the following results:

	Patients	Successes
Atrial tachysystole	3	2
Atrial extrasystole	3	3
Ventricular extrasystoles	17	16
Bouts of tachycardia	3	3
First degree block	8	5
Second degree block	6	5

In addition, in forty patients with atrial fibrillation, DPH was given before electroconversion was attempted. In a similar group, forty patients were given a beta-blocking agent before cardioversion was attempted. A comparison of these two groups showed to the advantage of DPH.

In a laboratory study, the authors performed atrial pacing with variable rhythm on ten dogs previously intoxicated by digitalis, and observed the effect of DPH. In three of ten cases, they observed a shortening of the P-R interval without modification of rhythm. In another experiment, a ligature was placed on both branches of the left coronary artery, to create a ventricular dysrhythmia. When overdigitalization produced rhythm disturbances, DPH was remarkably efficient, and in nine of ten cases the arrhythmia disappeared during injection.

The authors note that DPH corrects the disturbances of both atrial and ventricular excitability without impairing or even favoring atrioventricular conduction.

MATHUR, WAHAL, SETH and HAZRA, *Journal of the Indian Medical Association* (1971),[1339] state that diphenylhydantoin, administered orally to eighty-five patients with a variety of cardiac arrhythmias, was effective in the treatment of ventricular ectopics, ventricular tachycardia and in the majority of cases with supraventricular tachycardia. It was not found effective in cases with atrial fibrillation and heart block. Doses of DPH, 100 mg q.i.d. orally, were found to be safe and effective with minimal side effects.

STONE, KLEIN and LOWN, *Circulation*, (1971),[1598] state that the efficacy of diphenylhydantoin in preventing recurrent ventricular tachycardia was studied in ten patients, nine of whom had had myocardial infarction. The authors found DPH ineffective.

KOCH-WESER, *Archives of Internal Medicine* (1972),[1224] found diphenylhydantoin less effective than procainamide for the suppression of ventricular ectopic activity and prevention of serious ventricular arrhythmias in hospitalized patients with acute myocardial infarction. The author suggested that a trial of DPH in ambulatory patients with coronary heart disease appears worthwhile because its long-term administration is tolerated well by most patients.

KEMP, *Journal of the American Geriatrics Society* (1972),[1214] studied the effect of diphenylhydantoin on ventricular ectopic rhythms. These arrhythmias were not caused by digitalis. DPH was given to five patients and five patients were given placebo.

For the first three weeks the dosage of DPH was 100 mg q.i.d. Then for maintenance therapy during the rest of the three-month study the dosage was reduced to 100 mg t.i.d. The numbers of premature ventricular contractions during a five-minute continuous EKG monitoring period were recorded before therapy, after three weeks of therapy, and after three months of therapy.

There was a marked reduction in the number of ventricular ectopic beats in the DPH group compared with the control group, and the beneficial results continued despite reduction in the dosage of DPH.

CONDUCTION

BISSETT, DE SOYZA, KANE and MURPHY, *The American Journal of Cardiology* (1974),[831] directly measured conduction in the His-Purkinje system in fourteen patients and found that diphenylhydantoin improved intraventricular conduction.

The authors state that in 1950 DPH was reported to correct experimental ventricular tachycardia produced by coronary arterial ligation, and in 1954 it was shown to be effective in abolishing ouabain-induced ventricular tachycardia in dogs. Subsequent clinical experience confirmed the antiarrhythmic properties of DPH and its value in the treatment of ventricular tachycardia and ventricular arrhythmias induced by digitalis.

The authors state that the purpose of their study was to determine the effect of DPH on intraventricular conduction in man. Utilizing the introduction of premature atrial beats, the relative refractory period of the His-Purkinje system and the functional refractory period of the atrioventricular (A-V) node were measured in fourteen patients before and after administration of DPH. Before infusion of DPH, His-Purkinje conduction delay occurred with right bundle branch block in nine patients, and with left bundle branch block in five patients. After infusion of DPH (5 mg/kg at a rate of 50 mg/min) the onset or degree of His-Purkinje delay was improved in all patients. In the nine pa-

tients, DPH reduced the relative refractory period of the His-Purkinje system to a value less than that of the functional refractory period of the A-V node, so that His-Purkinje conduction delay no longer occurred after DPH.

In the five patients, DPH also reduced the relative refractory period of the His-Purkinje system or altered the degree of aberrant conduction, or both.

The authors note that before the introduction of His-bundle recordings, early reports had suggested that DPH may have no effect on intraventricular conduction in man. The results of the present study significantly demonstrate that DPH does improve intraventricular conduction in man.

ANDERSON, DAVIS, DOVE and GRIGGS, *Neurology* (1973),[764] studied the effect of diphenylhydantoin on cardiac conduction in patients who suffered from myotonic dystrophy. They found that DPH was beneficial, not only for the myotonia, but also for cardiac conduction defects common in this disease.

In five of the eight patients treated with oral DPH the P-R interval was shortened by 5 to 35 msec. This was in marked contrast to quinine and procainamide. Quinine produced P-R interval prolongation in four of ten patients, and procainamide produced P-R interval prolongation in nine of ten patients.

The authors' studies indicate diffuse involvement of the His-Purkinje system in myotonic dystrophy. They note that studies by others in normal subjects have shown a depression of His-Purkinje conduction with procainamide and quinine, but not with DPH.

BENAIM, CHAPELLE and CHICHE, *Annales de Cardiologie et d'Angeiologie* (1972),[816] reported on fifteen patients with arrhythmia who were injected with doses of 5 to 10 mg/kg of diphenylhydantoin. Recordings of the His potential achieved during the therapeutic test showed that 1) the drug does not usually alter the frequency of the sinus node; 2) it definitely improves atrioventricular conduction. In fact, a shortening of the P-H interval was obtained eight times out of eleven in conducted sinus rhythmus; 3) in most cases it did not alter intraventricular conduction: H-V remained constant eleven times out of fifteen. In four cases, a depression in intraventricular conduction was noted with a lengthening of the H-V interval.

In conclusion, the authors emphasize how valuable diphenylhydantoin is in arrhythmias, where these are accompanied by atrioventricular conduction defects.

QUIRET, BENS, DUBOISSET, LESBRE and BERNASCONI, *Archives des Maladies du Coeur et des Vaisseaux* (1974),[1434] studied the cardiovascular effects of diphenylhydantoin in 105 patients. They state that DPH appears to have the following pharmacodynamic properties. It favors or in any case respects atrioventricular conduction as well as intraventricular conduction; it checks manifestations of atrial and/or ventricular hyperexcitability secondary to organic cardiopathy or an excess of digitalis; and it has little or no effect on sinoatrial automatism. When it is injected slowly in the customary doses, its hemodynamic effects are very slight and fleeting.

The authors conclude that DPH thus appears to be an original effective antiarrhythmic as shown by their clinical trial covering 105 patients.

DAMATO, BERKOWITZ, PATTON and LAU, *American Heart Journal* (1970),[935] showed that in thirteen patients diphenylhydantoin enhanced atrioventricular conduction (i.e., shortened the P-H interval) over various paced heart rates. Also DPH did not prolong intraventricular conduction as measured by H-Q interval.

These observations were made while studying His bundle activities with an electrode catheter technique. (See also Caracta, et al.).[884]

MYOCARDIAL INFARCTION

HANSEN and WAGENER, *Munchener Medizinische Wochenschrift* (1969),[1120] reported the effective use of diphenylhydantoin in the treatment of cardiac arrhythmias following myocardial infarction.

In fifty patients who had a fresh myocardial infarction, DPH was slowly injected intravenously with excellent tolerance. There was no evidence of a pronounced hypotensive effect. The duration of action of 125 mg of DPH administered intravenously was eight to ten hours.

The authors state that bradycardiac arrhythmia does not constitute a contraindication to DPH.

YANG, *Journal of the Kansas Medical Society* (1973),[1705] states, "When faced with an intractable ventricular tachycardia and bewildered by the failure of treatment, try diphenylhydantoin (DPH); it could be life saving."

The author reports on a case of intractable ventricular tachycardia following acute myocardial infarction. Procainamide, large doses of lidocaine, repeated DC countershock, and propranolol failed to convert this life threatening cardiac arrhythmia which was dramatically controlled with DPH. DPH abolished the persistent ventricular tachycardia, which was believed to be due to circus re-entry rather than digitalis intoxication; it also permitted continuous digitalization when digitalis was so critically needed.

ANGINA PECTORIS

TAYLOR, *Chest* (1974),[1611] reports the effectiveness of diphenylhydantoin in angina pectoris, based on a double-blind crossover study with sixteen patients. The patients had typical symptoms of angina pectoris including chest pain, discomfort and tightness, radiating to arm, neck or jaw, precipitated by exertion, emotion and cold, and accompanied by dyspnea.

No anti-anginal drug therapy, apart from glyceryl trinitrate, was taken in the two-week period prior to the trial. Patients were divided into two groups, one that had both positive exercise tests and more than five pains a week during the double-blind placebo period, and a second group that had either negative exercise tests or less than five pains per week during the double-blind placebo period. DPH, 100 mg three times daily, was given for two weeks, alternating with placebo for two weeks, for a total of four weeks.

The number of attacks and severity of attacks were recorded by each patient and the duration of pain[1] was timed by each patient while on placebo and DPH. EKGs with or without exercise and two-step testing to the point of dyspnea, fatigue, or chest pain were given. On exercise tolerance tests patients stopped on an average of fifteen percent sooner with DPH. The double-blind study showed that oral DPH used as a prophylactic significantly reduced the frequency and the severity of symptoms in patients with angina pectoris.[2]

[1]No significant differences were noted in initial pain but duration of pain was reduced. *Note:* This is consistent with the basic mechanisms findings that initial pain impulses are not interfered with by DPH, but that repetitive after-discharge impulses are eliminated or decreased by DPH.

[2]Relevant basic mechanism studies are the demonstration of an increase in coronary blood flow by Gupta, et al.,[496] the improvement in coronary blood flow in dogs by Nayler, et al.[402] and by Haft, et al.[1110] and the improved survival, with DPH, of pigs after coronary occlusion by Zeft, et al.[392] and by Kong, et al.[433] See also Davies.[945]

BERNSTEIN, GOLD, LANG, PAPPELBAUM, BAZIKA and CORDAY, *JAMA* (1965),[18] in reporting on the effectiveness of diphenylhydantoin in the treatment of recurrent cardiac arrhythmias, noted that it was also useful in the treatment of angina pectoris in a sixty-seven year old female who had angina pectoris for six years.

When DPH was administered, 100 mg, orally three times a day, there was a marked lessening in the frequency and severity of the episodes of angina, and the patient reported a concurrent decrease in the frequency of palpitations, and a decrease in need for nitroglycerin. Before DPH, she required twelve to sixty nitroglycerin tablets per week; with DPH, she required only zero to four tablets per month.

HYPOKALEMIA

O'REILLY and MACDONALD, *British Heart Journal* (1973),[1390] reported on the successful use of diphenylhydantoin in treating two cases of ventricular arrhythmia induced by hypokalemia.

The authors state that the effectiveness of DPH in suppressing a variety of ventricular arrhythmias is well established. Despite this they say little emphasis has appeared in the published reports on the effectiveness of DPH in the presence of hypokalemia. This is the more remarkable as both procainamide and quinidine prolong the Q-T interval and so must aggravate the underlying defect which predisposes to arrhythmias when the serum potassium is low.[1]

The authors state that DPH, which has a different action at the cellular level and does not prolong the Q-T interval, seems an obvious choice in such cases.

In concluding the authors emphasize the usefulness of DPH in the management of the notoriously resistant and malignant arrhythmias associated with hypokalemia, where the usual antiarrhythmic agents are at best ineffective and may even be dangerous.

[1]Hypokalemia results in below normal potassium in nerve and muscle cells. Relevant to the above paper is the fact that DPH has been demonstrated to counteract low potassium levels in cells. (See "downhill movement" of ions, Ref. 387, 728, 731, 843, 1025, 1225, 1379, 1418, 1642, 1662.)

CARDIOVERSION

CUAN-PEREZ and ORTIZ, *Archivos del Instituto de Cardiologia de Mexico* (1971),[923] found diphenylhydantoin effective in preventing recurrence of fibrillation after cardioversion.

The study included 230 cases. DPH was compared with quinidine and propranolol and the authors found DPH the drug of choice.

DPH and the other two drugs acted in similar fashion with regard to percentage of recurrence. However, the authors found DPH the drug of choice because no toxic complications were observed with it and this was not the case with quinidine and propranolol.

LINDE, TURNER and AWA, *Pediatrics* (1972),[1289] in a review, suggest that because of the increased risk in cardioversion following digitalis administration, cardioversion should be preceded by diphenylhydantoin (5 mg/kg) administered intravenously over ten minutes, monitoring the electrocardiogram and blood pressure.

HYPERTENSION

ROSE, WILLIAMS, JAGGER, LAULER and THORN, *Metabolism* (1969),[1480] in a detailed study of two cases, demonstrate that diphenylhydantoin had a regulatory effect on labile hypertension.

When DPH was given to two patients whose blood pressure was abnormally elevated, the blood pressure returned to the normal range and stayed in the normal range as long as DPH was continued. In one of the patients DPH was discontinued on two separate occasions and on each occasion his blood pressure rose to pretreatment abnormal levels. Both times, when DPH was reinstituted, the patient's blood pressure returned to the normal range.

Both of these patients had a paradoxical response to dexamethasone. The authors suggest that in patients of this type the regulation of corticotropin-releasing-factor may be critical in the control of hypertension.[1]

[1]The above study calls attention to the fact that further exploration of the therapeutic effect of DPH on hypertension is indicated. Also see Ref. 414 and 1282.

CEREBRAL BLOOD FLOW

SLOSBERG, *Mt. Sinai Medical Journal* (1970),[1560] reports on his eight years of experience with medical therapy for cerebrovascular insufficiencies.

The author discusses what he has found to be a simple and effective regimen for treating cerebrovascular insufficiencies of diverse origins. This method consists of the use of diphenylhydantoin in conjunction with carotid sinus therapy and support stockings.

He states that these simple measures avoid the risk of surgical intervention and the hazards of anticoagulants; and that if his observations in sixty-one patients over an eight-year period are confirmed by others, this procedure could be the method of choice.

In the series of sixty-one patients, most of whom were in their sixties and seventies, there were a variety of cerebrovascular insufficiencies. Among these were patients with occlusive disease of the neck arteries, occlusive disease of the intracranial arteries, hypoplastic arteries; vascular anomalies of the circle of Willis; patients with reaction to compression of the common carotid arteries or of the carotid sinus areas; and patients with postural hypotension. There were included patients who had been candidates for neck vascular surgery, anticoagulants, vasodilators, or no treatment at all.

The author states that this method of diphenylhydantoin, carotid sinus therapy and support stockings has been both applicable and safe in a heterogeneous group of cases of cerebrovascular insufficiency for a period of over eight years; and has been well tolerated in both the acute stages of the illness and the long-term follow-up.

DANIEL, *Geriatrics* (1970),[938] states that symptoms of confusion which are so common in the aged often are caused by underlying physical illness, frequently cardiac and respiratory disorders resulting in cerebral anoxia. He states that diphenylhydantoin is therapeutically useful in this group, yet it is often overlooked.[1]

Among the symptoms of confusion so common in the aged are: 1) disorientation, often not of person but in particular of time, place and space; 2) lack of attention and concentration; 3) fluctuation in state of consciousness; 4) memory loss, particulary of current events; 5) poor performance when tested on immediate retention and recall; and 6) impairment of conventional judgment.

The author states that although problems of insufficient cerebral blood flow are well known in the aged, direct measurement of cerebral blood flow is at best difficult. However, the author states that symptoms of insufficient cerebral blood flow are identifiable clinically. Among these symptoms are irritability, restlessness, mental confusion and sometimes severe depression. The author notes that after cerebrovascular accident the patient often has paresthesias and tingling. He states that DPH not only frequently gives relief from the paresthesias, but that mental symptoms also improve.

The author states experience has shown that the improving mental state of the patient on DPH is a reasonable guide to over-all improvement in cerebral function.

[1]Occasionally a study is directly relevant in two separate clinical areas. This study also appears under Thought, Mood and Behavior Disorders.

KENNEDY, ANDERSON and SOKOLOFF, *Neurology* (1958),[1216] report that cerebral blood flow was significantly increased by diphenylhydantoin in a group of four epileptic children tested.

The cerebral blood flow of four epileptic children was studied before and after treatment with DPH for one week using a modified nitrous oxide test. The authors found that the mean blood flow in these children increased with DPH from 85 to 102 cc per 100 gram per minute. Although the group studied was small, the authors found the increase to be statistically significant.[1]

[1]The above observations were part of a study in which the authors found that the mean cerebral blood flow in ten epileptics, with no medication, was significantly less than the mean cerebral blood flow of eleven normals, 91.6 vs. 106.3cc/100g./min.

CARDIOVASCULAR BASIC MECHANISMS

The basic mechanisms paper of Harris and Kokernot, in 1950,[141] led to the use of DPH in cardiology. Some basic mechanisms studies are so relevant that they are repeated here for the convenience of the reader.

HYPOXIA IN PURKINJE FIBERS OF THE HEART[1]

BASSETT, BIGGER and HOFFMAN, *The Journal of Pharmacology and Experimental Therapeutics*

(1970),[804] in a study in which thirteen isolated dog hearts were used, found that DPH protected canine Purkinje fibers in heart, during hypoxia.

Background: The authors call attention to recent reports that indicate that ventricular arrhythmias

[1]For other demonstrations of DPH's usefulness in hypoxia, see Anti-anoxic Effects of DPH, p. 66.

are encountered in a high percentage of cases of ischemia caused by coronary artery occlusion, and that the results of numerous experiments suggest that Purkinje fibers are involved in the genesis of many ventricular arrhythmias. Hypoxia, ischemia and release of potassium and other intracellular substances could disturb cardiac rhythm by altering the sensitivity of Purkinje fibers.

The authors note that DPH has been found effective in abolishing many induced ventricular arrhythmias in dogs, including those caused by tying off the anterior descending coronary artery, and in pigs DPH has been shown to increase the number of survivors after experimentally induced myocardial ischemia and infarction. DPH has widely been found effective in abolishing many arrhythmias in man, including those following myocardial infarction.

The authors, in an earlier study using microelectrode techniques, had found that DPH had a protective effect on the electrophysiologic properties of canine Purkinje fibers subjected to toxic conditions, namely those induced by ouabain, those induced by low temperature and those induced by excessive stretch.

Methods and Conclusions: In the present study with isolated dog hearts, the authors state that they were concerned with the effectiveness of DPH in helping cardiac tissues survive during low oxygen tension. To determine the effect of DPH, the Purkinje fiber preparation of the isolated heart was stimulated electrically at a constant rate, and the electrical responses were measured until optimal performance was established. Then hypoxia was induced by perfusion with a nitrogen-carbon dioxide mixture. This hypoxia resulted in a sharp reduction in electrical response. The authors found that DPH improved electrical response, as measured by phase zero V_{max}, during hypoxia. They also found that DPH improved electrical response, as measured by phase zero V_{max}, when the Purkinje fiber had already been depressed by hypoxia.

The authors conclude that DPH improves the normal function of Purkinje fibers against lowered oxygen. They also note that when the Purkinje fibers had been impaired by hypoxia, DPH transiently improved this condition.

The authors suggest that the protective and therapeutic action of DPH on Purkinje fiber may in part explain the effectiveness of DPH in suppressing arrhythmias caused by myocardial ischemia and hypoxia.[1]

[1]This demonstration of the protective effect by DPH in isolated Purkinje fibers, against anoxia, is a separate source of evidence that DPH protects against anoxia at the cell level. See also Pincus,[699] Hadfield,[1109] Becker and Podos,[812] and p. 66.

PROTECTION AGAINST ARRHYTHMIAS INDUCED BY A VARIETY OF AGENTS

SPERELAKIS and HENN, *American Journal of Physiology* (1970),[1580] studied the effect of DPH on membrane potentials of individual chick heart cells in tissue culture. This method of separating cells from their nerves has the advantage of showing the direct effect of DPH on single cells, in this case, heart cells.

DPH was found to prevent hyperexcitability caused by both strontium and electrical pulses. Although DPH was protective against these insults, it did not affect the normal function of heart cells with regard to resting potentials, nor the maximum rate of rise or duration of the action potentials (even in high concentrations such as 1.8×10^{-5} M).

SINGH, SINHA, RASTOGI, DUA and KOHLI, *Japanese Journal of Pharmacology* (1971),[1557] studied the antiarrhythmic effects of DPH, paramethadione and trimethadione in dogs. Arrhythmias were induced by means of aconitine, hydrocarbon-epinephrine and coronary ligation. These arrhythmias were of both central and peripheral origin, and DPH was protective against both.

In addition, the authors state that DPH was

effective against all types of arrhythmias, irrespective of the nature and site of their origin, possibly because of its membrane-stabilizing properties.

CURTIS, *University of Michigan Doctoral Thesis* (1971),[927] in a study of experimental atrial fibrillation in dogs reported that DPH was as effective as quinidine in terminating stable atrial fibrillation which followed hypertonic solution administration.

He also noted that DPH has been effective against other animal models of experimental atrial fibrillation.

The author notes that in man DPH has not often been reported effective in chronic atrial fibrillation, although paroxysmal atrial fibrillation is reported to be prevented.[1]

[1]The papers of Singh, et al. and Curtis, above, agree on the effectiveness of DPH in atrial fibrillation in animals. However, they point up that in man differences still exist in the literature on the degree of effectiveness of DPH in chronic atrial arrhythmias. Further clinical evidence should make for clarification. See also pages 39 and 42, Vol. I.

CORONARY BLOOD FLOW

GUPTA, UNAL, BASHOUR and WEBB, *Diseases of the Chest* (1967),[496] were the first to demonstrate that DPH increases coronary blood flow in dogs.

NAYLER, McINNES, SWANN, RACE, CARSON and LOWE, *American Heart Journal* (1968),[402] demonstrated, in dogs, that DPH increases the coronary blood flow and that DPH reduces myocardial oxygen consumption.

ZEFT, REMBERT, CURRY and GREENFIELD, *Cardiovascular Research* (1973),[1711] in a study examining coronary blood flow, found that in intact conscious dogs, with the heart rate uncontrolled, DPH (5 mg/kg) produced a mean increase of 61% in coronary blood flow. With the heart rate controlled by ventricular pacing, a similar dose of DPH produced a mean increase in coronary blood flow of 57%. There was no significant change in either aortic blood flow or peripheral vascular resistance.

The authors concluded that to date DPH is the only antiarrhythmic agent which has been shown to improve coronary blood flow.

ZEFT, WHALEN, RATLIFF, DAVENPORT and McINTOSH, *The Journal of Pharmacology and Experimental Therapeutics* (1968),[392] conducted a study to evaluate the hypothesis that DPH given prophylactically would be effective in preventing death from ventricular arrhythmias resulting from experimental myocardial infarction. The left anterior descending coronary artery of forty farm pigs was gradually occluded with an Ameroid constrictor. The farm pig was chosen because the coronary artery pattern of this animal is relatively constant and similar to that of man.

Almost twice as many control animals (eleven of twenty) expired as DPH treated animals (six of twenty). Although the sample was not large enough to be conclusive, the authors state that there is an indication that DPH used prophylactically increases the chance of survival in experimental myocardial infarction in pigs.

As a result of this experiment the authors suggest that consideration should be given to the use of DPH on a regular basis as a prevention of fatalities originating from coronary artery disorders.

CEREBRAL BLOOD FLOW

BALDY-MOULINIER, *European Neurology* (1971-2),[790] found that DPH protected against the effects of cerebral ischemia. This anti-anoxic effect of DPH was demonstrated in cats in which the blood flow to the brain was stopped by clamping the aorta.

When control animals had the aorta clamped for seven minutes there was definitive electrical silence, absence of adequate cerebral blood re-flow, and increase in cerebrospinal fluid potassium level. In contrast, animals pretreated with DPH had definitive electrical recovery, steady cerebral blood flow and absence of the rise of cerebrospinal fluid potassium.

The animals treated with DPH could be revived for as long as fifteen minutes after occlusion of the aorta. The animals not treated with DPH could only be revived within seven minutes of occlusion. (Seven and fifteen are mean values.)

CONDUCTION

WAX, WEBB and ECKER, *Surgical Forum* (1969),[1668] in a study titled "Myocardium Stabilization by Diphenylhydantoin," observed the effect of DPH on the resting potential and the action potential of ventricular heart muscle of the rat.

Intracellular microelectrodes were used to measure the electrical potentials of individual ventricular muscle fibrils. With DPH the resting potential plateau phase and the recovery period were both lengthened.

The authors note that these actions of DPH would stabilize the heart and would make the heart less susceptible to early reentry from circus mechanisms or other rapid aberrant stimuli.

KLEINFELD and STEIN, *Circulation* (1968),[1221] electrically stimulated both isolated canine Purkinje and ventricular fibers and studied the action potentials. They found that DPH decreased the effective refractory period of both fibers with the greater effect being in the Purkinje fiber.

BIGGER, WEINBERG, KOVALIK, HARRIS, CRANEFIELD and HOFFMAN, *Circulation Research*

(1970),[828] studied the effects of diphenylhydantoin on excitability and automaticity in the canine heart.

The authors report that DPH 1) shortened the refractory period, particularly of ventricular muscle; 2) increased the multiple response and fibrillation thresholds in atrium and ventricle; 3) had little effect on diastolic threshold; 4) slightly enhanced the conduction velocity in ventricular muscle that was stimulated either in diastole or in its relative refractory period; and 5) produced slight decreases in automaticity in the ventricular specialized conducting system *in vivo*.

Also, in reporting on clinical experience the authors state that their experience suggests that DPH differs from quinidine in its effect on fundamental electrophysiological processes in the human heart. DPH does not prolong the Q-R-S interval and shortens the Q-T interval. These observations indicate that the drug does not prolong intraventricular conduction and suggest that it shortens the refractory period.

CALCIFICATION (CARDIAC)

RETTURA, STAMFORD and SEIFTER, *Paper presented at Northeast Regional Meeting of American Chemical Society* (1973),[1454] conducted a controlled study of the effect of DPH in mice with predisposition to cardiac calcification. This calcification was enhanced by stress.

The authors found that DPH reversed the calcification process as determined grossly, microscopically and by chemical analysis. The authors suggest that this might be one mechanism by which DPH is effective in the prevention of cardiac arrhythmias.

PROTECTION AGAINST DIGITALIS TOXICITY

GOLDSTEIN, PENZOTTI, KUEHL, PRINDLE, HALL, TITUS and EPSTEIN, *Circulation Research* (1973),[1085] state that the efficacy of DPH in treating digoxin toxicity is well established. In reporting the results of an extensive study of isolated dog heart, the authors state that DPH, when added to digoxin enhances the inotropic benefits of digoxin.

The authors found that before digoxin toxic levels are reached, DPH ultimately produces greater increase in contractile force, greater potassium efflux and greater inhibition of sodium-potassium-ATPase activity. The authors suggest that these are mechanisms which enable DPH to enhance the inotropic benefits of digoxin.[1]

[1]Although it is well established that DPH does not impair the inotropic benefits of the cardiac glycosides, we believe that this is the first paper to suggest that it may actually enhance the inotropic benefits of digoxin.

HANSEN and WAGENER, *Zeitschrift fur Kardiologie und Angiologie* (1974),[1122] by using both isolated atrium and barbiturate-damaged heartlung preparations of guinea pigs, showed that the toxic arrhythmic side effects of digoxin are prevented by DPH, without affecting its inotropic benefits. By the addition of DPH, glycoside dosages can be beneficially increased.

The authors conclude that DPH offers new aspects for the treatment of cardiac failure.

SCHERLAG, HELFANT, RICCIUTTI and DAMATO, *American Journal of Physiology* (1968),[1507] demonstrated in dogs that DPH consistently converted digitalis-induced ventricular tachycardia to sinus rhythm with a corresponding reversal of the digitalis-induced potassium efflux.

At the same time that the toxicity of digitalis was markedly delayed by DPH and the rate of myocardial potassium efflux slowed, the improvement in myocardial contractility with digitalis was not altered by DPH.

BASKIN, DUTTA and MARKS, *British Journal of Pharmacology* (1973),[801] in a study of the guinea pig heart, showed that DPH and potassium significantly prevent ouabain intoxication without preventing the inotropic benefits of ouabain.

WATSON and WOODBURY, *Archives Internationales de Pharmacodynamie et de Therapie* (1973),[1663] studying ouabain intoxication in guinea pigs, observed that DPH prevented ouabain induced electrolyte changes and prevented the development of ouabain-induced arrhythmias. Under some conditions, pretreatment with DPH reduced the lethality of ouabain from 90% to 34%. The authors concluded that these results are consistent with the concept that the antiarrhythmic effect of DPH is due to an action on active transport of electrolytes across cell membranes, since the plasma potassium was normalized by DPH pretreatment.

In addition, the authors measured the intracellular concentration of sodium, potassium and chloride in cardiac muscle and again observed a normalizing effect of DPH pretreatment.

Treatment of Pain

SUMMARY

The effectiveness of DPH in a variety of painful conditions is reviewed in The Broad Range of Use of DPH, Vol. I. Among these are the cranial nerve neuralgias including trigeminal neuralgia and glossopharyngeal neuralgia,[1] peripheral nerve neuralgias including polyneuritis, syphilitic and diabetic neuralgias,[2] migraine headache,[3] post-operative pain,[4] phantom limb pain,[5] pain of skeletal muscle spasms and of smooth muscle spasms.[6]

In recent studies, summaries of which follow, DPH is reported to be useful against other painful conditions. These are the pain of Fabry's disease, thalamic pain, angina pectoris, painful touching syndrome (dysesthesia), post-herpetic neuralgia, postsympathectomy neuralgia and pain of Wallenberg syndrome. Included elsewhere in this volume is found the effect of DPH on the pain of muscle spasms in myokymia[7] and multiple sclerosis.[8]

Initial messages of pain are necessary protective mechanisms. DPH does not interfere with initial electrical impulses.[9] However, when the usefulness of the initial messages of pain has ceased, persisting repetitive electrical impulses can occur (post-tetanic after-discharge). DPH reduces or abolishes post-tetanic after-discharge.[10] This seems to be an important mechanism by which DPH achieves its effect against pain.

DPH has general properties which enhance its usefulness in the treatment of pain.

1. DPH is not a sedative. In therapeutic doses, it does not slow cognitive and motor functions, as do many other substances used for pain.

2. DPH is not habit-forming. If it is necessary to use habit-forming substances for pain, smaller amounts of these substances may be used in conjunction with DPH.

[1] Ref. 9, 14, 15, 16, 31, 54, 68, 81, 113, 160, 175, 180, 202, 214, 224, 317, 330, 384, 518, 543, 583, 605, 611.

[2] Ref. 48, 129, 386.

[3] Ref. 40, 78, 111, 112, 113, 161, 227, 235, 315, 329, 338, 380, 420, 422, 429, 551, 587, 693, 748.

[4] Ref. 732, 744, 747.

[5] Ref. 704.

[6] Ref. 3, 66, 114, 304, 330, 429, 465, 551, 564, 586, 727.

[7] Ref. 633, 881, 1171, 1501, 1657, 1658, 1676.

[8] Ref. 304, 429, 586, 1192, 1242, 1243, 1342, 1360, 1541.

[9] Lack of interference with initial electrical impulses or other normal transmission, Ref. 90, 257, 289, 365, 458, 472, 954, 955, 1197, 1198, 1291, 1400, 1469, 1494, 1602.

[10] Ref. 90, 257, 264, 289, 359, 365, 458, 462, 467, 468, 472, 480, 580, 582, 789, 953, 954, 955, 1197, 1198, 1291, 1343, 1400, 1435, 1467, 1469, 1494, 1567, 1602, 1696.

PAIN IN FABRY'S DISEASE

LOCKMAN, HUNNINGHAKE, KRIVIT and DESNICK, *Neurology* (1973),[1299] based on a double-blind study, report the effectiveness of DPH in the relief of the pain of Fabry's disease, a rare disorder (see description below).[1]

The authors state that the single most debilitating and morbid aspect of Fabry's disease is the pain; this consists of two types, crises and continuous discomfort. Excruciating crises of abdominal, chest and muscle pain, as well as arthralgias and fever may occur episodically. These acute episodes occur periodically and may last several days. Many patients also complain of almost continuous discomfort. This second type of pain is initially noted in the fingers and toes and is characterized by a burning quality accompanied by paresthesias.

Since DPH has been reported to be useful in relieving pain associated with a variety of disease processes, the authors administered DPH to two patients with Fabry's disease. During this brief trial with DPH, both patients reported remission of their pain. As a result of the apparent relief of pain in these two patients, a double-blind crossover study with eight patients was done to more carefully evaluate the pain-relieving efficacy of DPH in Fabry's disease.

The medications compared were DPH, aspirin, and a multi-vitamin used as a placebo. The treatment period consisted of nine weeks with three-week treatment with each substance. The study was double-blind, with crossover, and patients were randomly assigned to six possible sequences of administration for the three substances. Adults received 300 mg of DPH daily; younger patients less. The daily dose of aspirin was 1800 mg per day.

Physical examinations as well as laboratory examinations were performed at the beginning and end of these studies, and in three cases trihexosyl ceramide determinations were performed.

The degree of pain relief experienced with each medication was monitored by having the patient complete daily diary sheets collected at weekly intervals. The study was completed by all patients, and the diaries were analyzed before the code for the medication was broken. The patients were asked to rate the relief of pain on a scale of 0 to 3: 1 representing fair relief; 2, good relief; and 3, complete relief.

The average relief score during DPH administration for all patients was 2.7 compared with the maximum possible score of 3.0. The pain relief score for aspirin was 0.5, and multi-vitamin, 0.9, respectively. The difference in relief between DPH and either of the other two substances was statistically significant (less than 0.001), whereas the difference in relief between aspirin and multi-vitamins was not significant.

The authors note that the pain in Fabry's disease is unrelieved by salicylates and it is only partially relieved by narcotics at soporific doses. The authors state that in the three cases in which trihexosyl ceramide levels had been determined no demonstrable change occurred. They therefore suggest that DPH's effectiveness in eliminating the debilitating pain of Fabry's disease is due primarily to its action on the nervous system.

---

[1]An X-linked inborn error of glycosphingolipid metabolism resulting from the deficient activity of ceramide trihexosidase, a specific alpha-galactosidase. The clinical manifestations are the result of the multisystemic accumulation of the glycosphingolipid substrate, trihexosyl ceramide, and include the characteristic cutaneous vascular lesions (angiokeratoma corporis diffusum), severe episodes of excruciating pain, and corneal opacities.

THALAMIC PAIN

CANTOR, *British Medical Journal* (1972),[883] reports that in two patients with thalamic pain, both experienced good relief with diphenylhydantoin.

The author states that the treatment of the painful, burning dysesthesias which can occur after thalamic infarction has been a particularly vexing problem, in that a variety of drugs have been tried with variable but generally ineffective results.

The author notes, with references to the literature, that relief of severe persistent pain by DPH has been reported in cases of trigeminal neuralgia, sphenopalatine neuralgia, tabes, and peripheral neuropathy. He also notes that in laboratory studies DPH has been shown to stabilize electrolyte transfer across neuronal membranes and to increase the neuronal threshold to repetitive stimulation; hyperexcitability is lessened by a reduction of both posttetanic facilitation and the duration of the afterdischarge following suprathreshold stimulation; and cortical responses to single repetitive thalamic stimulation are also reduced by DPH.

In light of both the clinical and laboratory findings it seemed reasonable to the author to postulate that DPH might be effective in thalamic pain by reducing the spread of abnormally excessive excitatory discharges resulting from the thalamic lesion.

The author reports that in each of the cases, when DPH treatment was stopped, the painful dysesthesia recurred. Reinstitution of DPH again resulted in alleviation of the pain.

Angina Pectoris

TAYLOR, *Chest* (1974),[1611] in a double-blind crossover study with sixteen patients, found that DPH used prophylactically reduced the frequency and severity of the pain of angina pectoris.[1]

[1]For more detailed summary see Cardiovascular Disorders, p. 27.

Dysesthesia (Painful Touching)

GERZ, *Physicians' Drug Manual* (1972),[1066] reports on an unusual case of "painful touching" (dysesthesia) in which a patient showed dramatic response to diphenylhydantoin.

The patient, a forty-year-old male, reported that a painful intolerable cold stream would run all over his body when being touched by human hand. He had once been married for two weeks, but the marriage was not consummated, since both partners had to sleep in separate bedrooms because of his refusal to be touched. Since being touched caused him

frequently to become dangerous and violent, he wanted a certificate from the clinic stating that he suffered from a "mental problem."

The patient presented a considerable diagnostic problem. He refused to have an EEG because of the extreme pain upon being touched. He was tried on a variety of medications without success.

Finally the patient was tried with DPH, 100 mg t.i.d. Within two weeks he was completely free of disturbing symptoms. Two months after taking DPH he joyfully reported that he had a girl friend and was now getting "the best things in life."

Neuralgias

HALLAQ and HARRIS, *Journal of American Osteopathic Association* (1969),[1116] report the successful use of diphenylhydantoin in a case of postherpetic neuralgia, with motor paralysis of an extremity, a rare complication. The patient, a seventy-six-year-old woman, had persistent pain in the right upper extremity, causing the entire limb to assume a semi-flexed and adducted position. Diagnosis after examination was postherpetic right brachial neuralgia and monoparesis.

After the seventh day in the hospital the patient was placed on DPH, 300 mg t.i.d. Within three days she was free of pain and remained free of pain when narcotic analgesics were withdrawn and an extra 100 mg of DPH was added.

With the relief of pain it became possible to institute vigorous rehabilitative and manipulative measures. Thirteen days after institution of DPH, 25% of lost functions were restored. The patient became an outpatient on a regimen of DPH and therapeutic exercises. A month later re-evaluation showed further improvement in function. The patient continued free of pain as long as she took DPH.

RASKIN, LEVINSON, PICKETT, HOFFMAN and FIELDS, *American Journal of Surgery* (1974),[1444] report on fifty-six patients who had had lumbar sympathectomy. Forty-four percent of these patients developed postsympathectomy neuralgia. Leg pain of these patients persisted one to two weeks. In some of them, the leg pain was described as a dull, deep ache in the anteromedial thigh. Aspirin or codeine were required by almost all patients who experienced this pain.

Eleven of the patients had pain of such great magnitude that they did not respond to meperidine. Carbamazepine was used with good effect in nine of these patients.

In two patients, intravenous diphenylhydantoin was used. Immediate relief from pain was experienced.

The authors conclude that DPH and carbamazepine appear to be useful in the management of the pain of the postsympathectomy syndrome.

PAIN IN WALLENBERG SYNDROME

MLADINICH, *JAMA* (1974),[1369] reports success in the use of diphenylhydantoin for relief of facial pain associated with Wallenberg syndrome. The author notes that the Wallenberg or posterior inferior cerebellar artery syndrome is the most common of the recognized brain stem "stroke" syndromes. Typical sequelae to cerebral thrombosis in the lateral medullary region of the brain stem are dysphagia, dysarthria, dysphonia, ipsilateral facial pain and hypalgesia, contralateral extremity hypalgesia, and ipsilateral incoordination.

A forty-year-old man, who had developed this syndrome two years previously, had been afflicted with ipsilateral burning facial pain around the eye. Ordinary analgesics did not relieve this pain, and he came to the hospital to seek relief. Because of the value of DPH in some pain syndromes, the author tried DPH, 1 gm in divided doses the first day and then 300 mg daily. Symptoms of facial pain were considerably relieved within several days, and in follow-up he continued to be relatively free of pain.

In discussing the use of DPH for the pain of the Wallenberg syndrome, the author notes that because facial pain can be a persistent and disabling symptom of the Wallenberg or posterior inferior cerebellar artery syndrome, a trial of DPH is recommended.

Muscle Disorders

SUMMARY

The effectiveness of diphenylhydantoin in continuous muscle fiber activity is observed clinically and demonstrated by quantitative electrophysiology.

In almost all of the cases which follow, a variety of medication had been used with little or no effect before the use of DPH.[1] Clinical recovery following the use of DPH was usually prompt; and on withdrawal of DPH relapse was also prompt.

Electromyographic tests demonstrate the electrical abnormality in these disorders before the use of DPH and demonstrate correction of this abnormality with DPH. This provides evidence, in muscle, as in other areas, that DPH corrects inappropriate electrical activity such as post-tetanic after-discharge and dysrhythmias.

The studies which follow are so detailed that they do not lend themselves to summary form. For this reason, with the exception of the earliest reported work, that of Isaacs, only brief descriptions will be given—the reader is referred to the full papers.

There are many symptoms in common in continuous muscle fiber activity disorders, and there are also differences. These differences are reflected in the wide variety of terminology used by the authors. Although the terminology differs, the disorders have much in common. They are the cause of much suffering, are disabling, and frequently incapacitating.

[1]Later, in some of the cases carbamezapine was also found effective.

CONTINUOUS MUSCLE FIBER ACTIVITY

The following report, by Isaacs, is believed to be the first publication of the successful use of diphenylhydantoin in the treatment of continuous muscle fiber activity syndrome.

ISAACS, *Journal of Neurology, Neurosurgery and Psychiatry* (1961),[176] in a study entitled "Continuous Muscle Fiber Activity" describes this disorder in a twelve-year-old boy.

This twelve-year-old boy walked with extreme difficulty, in a rigid manner. All his muscles showed evidence of fasciculation and were weak. The weakness particularly affected the extensor muscles of the forearms, arms, extensor and peroneal muscles of the legs, and the small muscles of the hands and feet. He was constantly covered with a thin film of perspiration, had a persistent tachycardia and slight fever. Upper limbs could only be fully extended passively and then with difficulty. Electrocardiograms appeared normal. However, electromyography recorded a state of constant rapid dysrhythmic discharge of independent muscle fibers. The spontaneous activity was increased by voluntary contraction, an increase which persisted for 30± seconds after the stimulus had ceased.

The author defines the state as myotonic after-discharge and likens it to post-tetanic after-discharge.

Medications tried without success. The patient showed no improvement following the administration of quinidine, procainamide, cortisone or potassium depletion by exchange resins. Each of these was given for periods of at least a month and doses pushed to the point of maximum tolerance. Short-lived improvements followed injections of Dimercaprol.

Course of illness. Over the next two years the patient was further investigated whenever possible. His condition appeared static. Splints were made and applied at night to prevent flexion deformities of elbows and wrists and to counteract the developing pes cavus. Growth remained retarded, muscle bulk had diminished, and he had brief attacks of acute respiratory embarrassment due to chest and diaphragmatic stiffness.

Successful treatment with DPH. By this time, Isaacs had successfully used diphenylhydantoin with another patient. As a result of this success, the twelve-year-old boy was brought back to the hospital and treated with DPH. The author states that his recovery was dramatic.

The second case of continuous muscle fiber activity, just referred to, was that of a fifty-three-year-old male.

Medications tried without success. The patient had been treated with atropine, quinine, cortisone, artane, adenosine triphosphate, thiamine diphosphate and procainamide without effect.

Course of illness. The patient's condition steadily deteriorated for over a year, so that he became unable to walk and began developing contractures in the upper and lower limbs, producing flexion deformities at the elbows and wrists and pes cavus respectively. There were several episodes of respiratory embarrassment and dysphagia.

Successful treatment with DPH. Diphenylhydantoin was used in an attempt to diminish the bizarre uncontrolled discharge in the lower motor neuron which characterizes this condition. The author had exhausted the possibilities of deficient or excessive ions concerned in the maintenance of normal neuromuscular response, and had abandoned both blocking and depolarizing agents as therapeutic tools owing to the occurrence of severe muscle weakness.

The initial dose of DPH was 100 mg every four hours. A marked improvement occurred over the next two days and the dose was reduced to 100 mg q.i.d.

The electromyography was vastly improved both at rest and on voluntary effort. The B.M.R. was +7, and the oxygen consumption had fallen to 280 ml./minute after only two weeks of DPH therapy.

Follow-up. In a follow-up of the two patients five years later, Isaacs[1183] reports that both patients were still well, had lost their abnormal stiffness and live fairly normal lives. He also notes that whenever DPH has been stopped, the symptoms have returned.[1]

In a later paper titled "Quantal Squander,"[177] the author postulates that the problem in continuous muscle fiber activity may lie with the acetylcholine quantal release mechanism.

[1]The author later observed that carbamezapine could be used as a substitute for or in combination with DPH but states that the patients preferred DPH.

ISAACS, *Journal of Neurology, Neurosurgery and Psychiatry* (1967),[1183] reports on another patient with continuous muscle fiber activity, a twenty-year-old Indian male. The rapid effectiveness of diphenylhydantoin was apparent. DPH, 100 mg q.i.d., enabled this patient to return to an almost normal state, within three days.

In discussing the basic physiological problem in this disorder, Isaacs notes that normal muscle is virtually electrically silent until contraction is initiated. In myotonia, however, during relaxation, the clinical problem becomes apparent because, as the author points out, this is when the myotonic after-discharge occurs.[1]

[1]The stabilization of myotonic after-discharge is a demonstration of the property of DPH to stabilize a hyperexcitable condition as in post-tetanic potentiation and post-tetanic after-discharge. (See Ref. 90, 257, 289, 365, 458, 467, 468, 472, 789, 954, 955, 1197, 1198, 1291, 1343, 1400, 1467, 1469, 1494, 1602.)

MERTENS and ZSCHOCKE, *Klinische Wochenschrift* (1965),[251] in a paper entitled "Neuromyotonia" report on three cases. Each patient had in common a continuous spastic contraction of the entire skeletal musculature, which did not even diminish while asleep or under anesthesia. Extensive electromyographic, histologic and other laboratory studies confirmed the electrophysiological abnormality. Quinine, quinidine, novocamid, cortical hormones and saldiuretics had little or no effect.

Diphenylhydantoin and Mephenytoin were tried. DPH was far more effective. With two injections of DPH, 250 mg, at sixty-minute intervals it was possible to obtain significant elimination of spastic contractions and inhibition of movement in all muscle groups within two to four hours.

The authors state that with oral DPH they were able to maintain this astonishing effect. A trial of discontinuing the DPH resulted in recurrence or rapid increase of the abnormal contraction. Later carbamezapine was used with similar effectiveness on these patients.

LEVY, WITTIG and FERRAZ, *Arquivo de Neuro-Psiquiat* (1965),[1280] in a paper entitled "Scleroderma Associated with Continuous Muscular Electrical Activity" described a case, difficult to diagnose, in which clinical examination and laboratory tests indicated probable scleroderma. However, there was a definite condition of continuous muscle fiber activity at rest, revealed by electromyography. The condition showed some clinical improvement with corticosteroids, although this improvement was not reflected on the electromyogram.

The authors expressed surprise at the results of the use of 300 mg of DPH daily because of its speed in markedly improving both the clinical picture and the abnormal electrical tracing in a few days.

HUGHES and MATTHEWS, *Journal of Neurology, Neurosurgery and Psychiatry* (1969),[1171] in a paper entitled "Pseudo-Myotonia and Myokymia" report on a man whose symptoms had gradually worsened from the age of twenty-two. When seen he was fifty-five. Electromyography demonstrated the patient's electrical abnormality. He had been tried on a variety of substances without benefit.

Thirty-two years after the first symptoms had been noted he was treated with 100 mg of diphenylhydantoin q.i.d. This produced immediate and continuing benefits. The patient found that he could control the stiffness adequately with 200 to 300 mg of DPH daily, although fasciculation continued and delayed relaxation of grip could still be detected. The patient noticed that if he stopped taking DPH for as short a period as twenty-four hours the symptoms would return.

Five years after the institution of DPH, carbamezapine was also tried and found effective. The patient seemed to prefer carbamezapine, but the author states that he failed to find any convincing difference in the response to the two medications.

GARDNER-MEDWIN and WALTON, *Lancet* (1969),[633] in a paper entitled "Myokymia with Impaired Muscular Relaxation," describe a twenty-one-year-old female who had suffered with this disorder for about four-and-a-half years. This patient had characteristic clinical and electromyographic evidence of myokymia, and had had operations on her tendons with only temporary relief.

The patient was treated with diphenylhydantoin,

100 mg t.i.d., and diazepam, 5 mg twice daily. On this treatment the patient improved considerably and was able to lead a relatively normal life.

WALLIS, VAN POZNAK, and PLUM, *Archives of Neurology* (1970), [1658] in a paper entitled "Generalized Muscular Stiffness, Fasciculations and Myokymia of Peripheral Nerve Origin" report on two cases with this disorder. Electromyographic and other laboratory findings were consistent with the clinical diagnosis.

In one case the authors state diphenylhydantoin, 100 mg t.i.d., provided dramatic relief. In the other case a three-day trial with DPH was not found effective. In the successful case, after one month of treatment, the DPH was discontinued, and three days later all pretreatment symptoms and findings had returned. With the reinstitution of DPH prompt relief recurred, and this has lasted for eight months to the present writing. This patient had been severely incapacitated and has returned almost to normal.

BUSCAINO, CARUSO,, DE GIACOMO,, LABIANCA and FERRANNINI, *Acta Neurologica* (1970), [881] in a paper entitled "Unusual Neuromuscular Pathology" describe a case of continuous muscle fiber activity syndrome (neuromyotonia).

The man, age forty-five, had suffered for twenty years from stiffness of all muscles, wide-spread fasciculations, myokymia and excessive sweating. The muscular stiffness was present even during sleep. The nature of the electrical abnormality in this disorder was observed on the electromyogram.

This condition, present for twenty years, had been treated with a variety of substances without success. The authors state that the condition was dramatically resolved by the use of diphenylhydantoin or carbamezapine.

WELCH, APPENZELLER and BICKNELL, *Neurology* (1972), [1676] in a study entitled "Peripheral Neuropathy with Myokymia, Sustained Muscular Contraction and Continuous Motor Unit Activity" describe a twenty-two-year-old female who over the years had had gradually increasing symptoms of this disorder. The patient's symptoms included stiffness and weakness of the upper arms and shoulders and proximal lower extremities, dysarthric speech and occasional labored respiration because of tightness of the chest wall. The electromyograph showed continuous motor unit action potentials. Microscopic examination of the sural nerve showed evidence of peripheral neuropathy.

The patient was tried with quinine regularly for one month but no change in symptoms was noted. Then the patient was given diphenylhydantoin, 100 mg before noon and 200 mg at bedtime, with almost immediate remission of the symptoms. This remission continued with daily DPH.

KOSTOV, TACHEV and NASTEV, *Zhurnal Nevropatologii i Psikhiatrii imeni S.S. Korsakova* (1973), [1231] in a paper entitled "Pseudo-Myotonia (Isaacs' Syndrome)" report on a case with a form of this syndrome characterized by muscular hypertonia mainly expressed in the distal regions of the extremities. Diffuse fascicular tics were present. Spontaneous electromyographic activity was present at rest, and typically did not disappear even after novocain blockade of the peripheral nerve.

Diphenylhydantoin and carbamezapine each had favorable therapeutic effect. Withdrawal of the medications resulted in a return of the disorder.

BHATT, VIJAYAN and DREYFUS, *California Medicine* (1971), [825] in a review of clinical and laboratory aspects of myotonia, state that of treatments which have been used successfully for myotonia, including diphenylhydantoin, procainamide, quinine, and adrenocorticotropic hormone, DPH appears to be the most effective, the safest and the best tolerated.

MUNSAT, *Neurology* (1967), [262] in a randomized, double-blind and crossover study, found diphenylhydantoin to be as effective as procainamide in relieving myotonia, both subjectively and objectively.

The author stated that DPH was better tolerated by patients than procainamide and, in addition, unlike procainamide, it did not increase preexisting cardiac conductive defects.

THOMPSON, *New England Journal of Medicine* (1972), [1614] in a letter to the editor wrote:

"Therapy of myotonia with diphenylhydantoin was reported by T.L. Munsat in Neurology (17:359, 1967). However, there has been little published in the literature to support or contradict his studies.

In three members of a family in my practice with myotonia congenita, diphenylhydantoin, 100 mg three times a day, was started on April 29, 1971. The patients were 16 (female), 20 (female) and 23 (male) years of age. Their disabilities included inability to dance, difficulty getting up from a sitting position, difficulty relaxing grips, and some falling because of inability to relax the muscles.

On diphenylhydantoin therapy they are all much improved. The 16-year-old girl is particularly delighted because she can now dance. No side effects have occured and the improvement is dramatic."

The writer says that certainly other patients with myotonia should be given the benefits of diphenylhydantoin.

GIMENEZ-ROLDAN and ESTEBAN, *European Neurology* (1973), [1073] reported a case of myotonia associated with hypothyroidism in which diphenylhydantoin and quinine sulfate was rapidly effective for some but not all of the symptoms.

ANDERSON, DAVIS, DOVE and GRIGGS, *Neurology* (1973), [764] studied the effect of diphenylhydantoin on cardiac conduction in patients who suffered from myotonic dystrophy. They found that DPH was beneficial, not only for the myotonia, but also for cardiac conduction defects common in this disease.

In five of the eight patients treated with oral DPH the P-R interval was shortened by 5 to 35 msec. This was in marked contrast to quinine and procainamide. Quinine produced P-R interval prolongation in four of ten patients, and procainamide produced P-R interval prolongation in nine of ten patients.

The authors' studies indicate diffuse involvement of the His-Purkinje system in myotonic dystrophy. They note that studies by others in normal subjects have shown a depression of His-Purkinje conduction with procainamide and quinine, but not with DPH.

The authors state that since they and others have found that DPH is an effective antimyotonic agent and since their own findings have shown that it does not have negative effects on conduction abnormalities as do quinine and procainamide, DPH is the treatment of choice in myotonic dystrophy.

CHOREOATHETOSIS

TASSINARI and FINE, *Proceedings of the Australian Association of Neurologists* (1969), [1610] give the history of a patient with paroxysmal choreoathetosis, a twenty-three-year-old man, complaining of episodes of uncontrollable involuntary movements since the age of eleven. The writhing flinging movements in this patient were of such intensity that sometimes the patient was thrown to the floor. The attacks were most frequent in childhood and followed an irregular pattern. There were good days and there were bad days. In the latter, there could be ten to thirty attacks a day.

The patient was treated with diphenylhydantoin, 100 mg t.i.d., and Valium, 5 mg t.i.d. With this treatment the frequency and intensity of attacks were reduced to once or twice a week and never severe enough to cause a fall, and the patient resumed a normal social life. On the two occasions that the treatment was interrupted, there followed a reappearance of attacks as frequent and severe as before treatment.

JUNG, CHEN and BRODY, *Neurology* (1973),[1200] report on ten cases of paroxysmal choreoathetosis in two families. They also report on two sporadic cases. The authors state that to their knowledge this is the first report of its occurrence among the Chinese. The authors state that the onset of this disorder usually appears in childhood with sudden brief and intermittent choreoathetoid movements of the extremities and face. Episodes may occur several times daily with varying degrees of bizarre posturing, which can reach such intensity that the patient is hurled to the floor. Consciousness is not lost. With age these attacks tend to diminish in frequency and severity, and this sometimes makes it more difficult to evaluate the effectiveness of drugs.

The authors state that the therapeutic effect of diphenylhydantoin is so prompt and so dramatic that there is little doubt as to the effectiveness of the treatment. They state that except for one early report, DPH has been the drug of choice for this disorder.

LOONG and ONG, *Journal of Neurology, Neurosurgery and Psychiatry* (1973),[1305] reported a case of a twenty-one-year-old Chinese man whose choreoathetosis was successfully treated with diphenylhydantoin. Daily attacks of muscle spasms, involving the right limbs predominantly, had occurred up to twenty times a day for two years. Chlordiazepoxide and amitriptyline produced no improvement. DPH 100 mg t.i.d. was effective in completely freeing the patient of "big" attacks, and "small" ones occurred only a few times a day. L-dopa was also effective in this case. When DPH was withdrawn the symptoms returned, and when DPH was reinstituted, the improvement again occurred.

OTHER MUSCLE DISORDERS

STEROID MYOPATHY

STERN, GRUENER and AMUNDSEN, *JAMA* (1973),[1594] treated a forty-seven-year-old man with steroid myopathy with diphenylhydantoin with favorable results. The myopathy was well documented and the effectiveness of DPH was demonstrated by a double-blind crossover method.

The patient required steroids (prednisolone) for his rheumatoid arthritis. Without changing the regimen of prednisolone, two six-week trial periods of DPH and placebo capsules were instituted with crossover every three weeks. The results of the two trials revealed that while on DPH there was a significant improvement as measured by increase in hip flexor strength as contrasted to placebo. Muscle strength was measured with a dynamometer.

The authors state that although this was only one case, the results are encouraging because they suggest that DPH, when used along with steroids, may decrease the risk of steroid myopathy. (See Gruener and Stern,[1103] DPH protection against steroid myopathy in mice. See Houck, et al.,[172,501,502] DPH protection against side effects of cortisone as observed in the skin of rats.)

RESTLESS LEGS

HOGG, *Practitioner* (1972),[1155] in a paper on "Restless Legs or Ekbom's Syndrome" describes the successful treatment of seven cases of "restless legs" with diphenylhydantoin. The author says that interest in this syndrome was renewed by Ekbom twenty-six years ago, but it was first described as far back as 1685. It is still a syndrome of unknown etiology. Vasodilators, iron intravenously and intravenous Dextran have been tried with only partial success.

The syndrome, he states, derives its name "restless legs" from the fact that the majority of these patients are unable to rest in bed at night and take to moving their legs sometimes vigorously because of the gnawing aches in them and the "crawling pains."

The author states that this syndrome can be seen in all age groups, but chiefly in pre-menopausal women. Frequently these patients suffer from depression or anxiety states.

The author gives brief descriptions of the seven cases:

Case 1. Age 73. This elderly man complained of cramp-like sensations in his groin which made him get out of bed and walk the floor after being in bed just a few minutes.

Case 2. A 33-year-old woman complained initially of colicky abdominal pains which were worse just before a period. She was depressed and complained that when she got into bed at night or sat in a chair for any length of time she had crawling sensations in the calves and had to walk for relief.

Case 3. A woman, 57 years old, was depressed and only reported restless legs on questioning as to how she slept at night.

Case 4. A man, age 60, had had angina pectoris for years, complained of restless legs which were worse in bed at night.

Case 5. A woman, age 45, had had a hysterectomy for heavy, frequent periods, and developed restless legs after the operation.

Case 6. A woman, 30 years old, a second pregnancy precipitated restless legs.

Case 7. Mrs. A. H., again a second pregnancy precipitated restless legs.

Results. In each of the seven patients, 100 mg of diphenylhydantoin daily resulted in cessation of symptoms. Since the symptoms occurred at night, and interrupted sleep, the 100 mg was given before going to bed.

PARKINSON'S SYNDROME

DOMZAL, *Neurologia i Neurochirurgia Polska* (1972),[971] reported on the use of diphenylhydantoin in treating fourteen patients exhibiting a complete clinical picture of Parkinson's syndrome. Eight of these patients had received synthetic anticholinergic drugs, and six had not received any previous anti-Parkinsonism medication. The clinical condition of these patients was evaluated according to four parameters, i.e., tremor, sluggishness, muscle tone and the patient's frame of mind.

With DPH, in doses of 300-400 mg per day over a two-week period, eleven patients reported marked improvement in sense of well-being; ten reported improvement in muscle tone; and six exhibited improvement in general tremor (tremor disappeared entirely in three). Steadier mobility, better expression and improved gait were observed in three patients.

The author says that it is apparent that DPH exerts a favorable effect on the clinical condition in some of the cases of Parkinsonism, appearing to be more effective in the initial stages of the disease. DPH affects the increase of muscle tone most favorably, but immobility, disturbances of posture, gait and speech are less affected.

The author stated that there are few drugs that can withstand the test of time and still continue to stir increasing interest; DPH, in particular, belongs in this category. He felt that the limited number of cases involved in his study did not permit him to offer any conclusions, but suggests that DPH may prove to be a valuable drug in the treatment of certain cases of Parkinson's disease.

MUSCLE SPASMS

SATOYOSHI and YAMADA, *Archives of Neurology* (1967),[1501] in a paper entitled "Recurrent Muscle Spasms of Central Origin" present two cases of painful intermittent muscle spasms of a slowly progressive nature. Each began in early life. Multiple bony abnormalities with epiphyseal destruction and retarded growth, diarrhea, disturbed carbohydrate metabolism and endocrine disorders were additional features. In both patients single oral doses of three grams of potassium chloride produced bouts of repetitive generalized spasms lasting for several days. The severity and frequency of the cramps was increased by the administration of acetazolamide, 500 mg, and hydrochlorothiazide, 50 mg. Numerous other drugs were given without effect on the spasms: calcium lactate, Vitamin D, magnesium sulphate, desoxycorticosterone, dexamethazone, hydrocortisone, prednisolone, diazepoxide, diazepam, neostigmine, mephenesin and phenobarbital.

Calcium gluconate with 10 percent glucose intravenously occasionally reduced the frequency and severity of the spasms, as did also quinine sulfate and procainamide.

Diphenylhydantoin (200 to 300 mg daily by mouth) was even more effective. This effectiveness was further evidenced by the fact that when the medicine was withdrawn the attacks would return. Combination of DPH, quinine sulfate and chlorpromazine was found to be the most beneficial. Even with this regimen muscle spasms could not be completely forestalled.

Later in 1967 a third case was presented by Satoyoshi[1502] in which he reports similar results.

MATTHEWS, *Brain* (1958),[1342] reported the effectiveness of diphenylhydantoin in the treatment of tonic seizures in a patient with multiple sclerosis. When DPH, 100 mg t.i.d. was prescribed, the attacks stopped within two days. Treatment was stopped after two months with no return of these symptoms. Other sensory and ataxic symptoms recurred later, characteristic of multiple sclerosis. It was not claimed by the author that DPH had any primary beneficial action on multiple sclerosis itself, but that it was found useful in the treatment of the painful spasms of this disorder.

JOYNT and GREEN, *Archives of Neurology* (1962),[1192] found that diphenylhydantoin had definite suppressing effects on tonic seizures in three patients with multiple sclerosis.

KUROIWA and SHIBASAKI, *Folia Psychiatrica et Neurologica Japonica* (1968),[1243] found that diphenylhydantoin and/or carbamazepine were useful in suppressing the painful tonic spasms in four patients with multiple sclerosis. The authors noted

that various other drugs (phenobarbital, diazepam, chlorpromazine, biperiden, procainamide, quinine hydrochloride, calcium gluconate and gamma-hydroxy beta-amino butyric acid) were tried in all four cases, but all without success.

The authors noted that the beneficial effects of DPH might relate to its known regulatory effects on spinal cord and peripheral nerves. They postulated that DPH may be counteracting an unusual excitation of a sensory-motor-neuronal complex and unusual transmission or conduction of the impulses in the affected spinal cord level or in the lower brain stem (see also Shibasaki and Kuroiwa).[1541]

HICCUPS

PETROSKI and PATEL, *Lancet* (1974),[1411] in a letter to the editor, report on a patient with refractory hiccups. On admission to the hospital, the patient, a thirty-seven-year-old man, had a three-year history of hypertension, an old right-hand hemiparesis and hiccups. He was mentally alert, but repetitive attacks of hiccups seriously interfered with his feeding and sleep and left him exhausted. The hiccups did not respond to pharyngeal stimulation by catheter or parenteral prochlorperazine, up to 50 mg per day, nor did the frequency vary with sleep. By the sixth day the frequency of hiccups increased to more than thirty per minute. On the hypothesis that an irritable focus in the area of the inspiratory center of the medulla might be occurring, diphenylhydantoin was started.

Initially 200 mg of DPH intravenously was given over five minutes, completely eliminating hiccuping within an hour. Then 100 mg. q.i.d. orally was continued until the eleventh day without any recurrence of hiccups.

DAVIS, *Lancet* (1974),[946] in a letter to the editor, stated that he was interested to read the report by Petroski and Patel on the use of DPH in treating hiccups. He states: "Unfortunately, in a patient with long-established hiccups with whom I have recently been concerned, this drug (DPH) was ineffective. Nevertheless, it should no doubt be added to the list of preparations to be considered in cases of intractable hiccup."

RESPIRATORY MYOCLONUS

PHILLIPS and ELDRIDGE, *New England Journal of Medicine* (1973),[1414] in a paper entitled "Respiratory Myoclonus (Leeuwenhoek's Disease)" describe a case of abnormal repetitive diaphragmatic contractions in which treatment with diphenylhydantoin either abolished or markedly reduced the abnormal activity. The authors state that these cases are sometimes called diaphragmatic flutter, and they suggest the term respiratory myoclonus could be appropriate.

The authors note that diphenylhydantoin had escaped previous reported clinical trial for this disorder. Because of its established effect on synapse and membrane stabilization they decided to try it on this patient. A dosage of 300 mg daily was not found effective, but at 400 mg daily the desired effect occurred. Improvement was noted after five or six days of therapy.

DPH was discontinued on three separate occasions with return of the disorder. A diaphragmatic electromyogram taken during DPH therapy, during quiet breathing, showed definite slowing of the respiratory rate.

More important was the absence of the alternating electrical bursts of activity and silence during inspiration, and the disappearance of abnormal activity during expiration. Identical desired effects were also demonstrated by electromyography in the scalene and intercostal muscles.

The authors state that a trial of quinidine to a maximum of three grams daily had been ineffective. At the time of the writing the patient had taken DPH daily for about a year with no recurrence of symptoms.

The authors note that in the past the only effective form of therapy for this disorder has been phrenicectomy. They state that therapy with DPH might be effective in some patients.

CASES IN WHICH DPH NOT FOUND USEFUL

Diphenylhydantoin was reported to not be useful in a case of post-stroke palatal myoclonus,[1462] a case of hereditary essential myoclonus,[942] a case of facial contraction in brain stem glioma,[1613] a case of congenital disorder of motor control,[1701] a case of involuntary movements associated with erythrocyte malformations,[922] and one of facial spasm associated with Paget's disease.[952] Twelve patients were reported not significantly helped with "irritable bowel syndrome."[1098]

Treatment of Other Disorders

SCLERODERMA

MORGAN, *Cutis* (1971),[1371] reports that patients with scleroderma, treated with DPH, showed marked improvement, in a study comparing them with patients treated by conventional therapy.

The study consisted of sixty-five patients with two general types of scleroderma, morphea and systemic. Twenty-nine were treated with DPH and thirty-six were treated by conventional means.

The author notes that no therapeutic measures advocated in the past have resulted in consistent improvement in scleroderma, although on occasion some symptoms and complications have shown response to a wide variety of substances.

The attention of the author was brought to the use of DPH in scleroderma in an unusual way. A sixty-seven-year-old woman had progressive generalized morphea with associated headaches, arthralgias, dysphagia, and palmar and plantar hyperhidrosis. For over a year numerous medications (including phenylbutazone, methysergide, diazepam, belladonna alkaloids, proteolytic enzymes, entozyme, DMSO, tocopherol, potassium p-aminobenzoate, ergotamine tartrate, steroids, and tolazoline) had failed to halt progression of the disease.

The patient had a mild stroke and as a result was placed on DPH by attending neurologists. Progressive improvement in scleroderma was evident three weeks after she began DPH therapy. Two years later her skin showed no evidence of scleroderma and has remained clear to date.

Because of the unexpected improvement in this case, the author decided to explore the possibility that DPH might be effective in the treatment of scleroderma. In his study the author used DPH in twenty-nine patients and conventional therapy in thirty-six patients. The results follow:

Number of Patients	With DPH 29	Other Therapy Or None 36
Worse	0 (0%)	11 (30.5%)
No change	2 (7%)	10 (28%)
Improved (patient and doctor agree)	12 (41.5%)	9 (25%)
Complete clearing of sclerosis	12 (41.5%)	4 (11%)
Complete clearing of sclerosis plus atrophy and pigment	3 (10%)	2 (5.5%)

The author concludes that in this series of patients with scleroderma, the administration of DPH not only appeared to prevent progression of sclerosis but to aid in its resolution. [1,2]

[1] In a smaller group of patients, the author also investigated the use of DPH in a less serious disorder, lichen sclerosis et atrophicus, and found DPH effective but, in this case, no more than conventional therapy.

[2] Of interest in connection with this study are both clinical and basic mechanisms studies which report other healing effects of DPH. (See Ref. 25, 127, 171, 172, 188, 189, 335, 336, 337, 339, 341, 343, 344, 499, 500, 501, 502, 504, 505, 669, 730, 811, 894, 1080, 1104, 1164, 1403, 1485, 1504.)

ASTHMA

SHAH, VORA, KARKHANIS and TALWALKAR, *Indian Journal of Chest Diseases* (1970),[1535] conducted a study of the usefulness of DPH in bronchial asthma in twenty-seven patients. Both clinical and laboratory observations were made.

The authors state that the prevention of the spread of electrical discharge is one of the most important, interesting and unexploited pharmacological properties of diphenylhydantoin. Noting that other paroxysmal disorders have responded to DPH, they felt that its use in the paroxysmal spasm of asthma should be explored.

In the study of the twenty-seven patients, careful histories were recorded, the severity of asthma was graded by age at onset, frequency of attacks during past twelve months, absenteeism from work, number of days absent in the last month, and number of sleepless nights in the last month. Effort tolerance tests were performed during attacks and between attacks. Appraisal of previous therapy during the last month was noted by the number of adrenalin and/or aminophylline injections and oral drugs—bronchodilators and/or steroids. Each patient had laboratory investigations, chest x-ray and electrocardiogram to exclude any cardiopulmonary disease simulating bronchial asthma. Ventilation studies, including maximum breathing capacity, were carried out initially and repeated at weekly follow-up examinations. At the end of the treatment period all examinations were repeated.

Before starting patients on DPH therapy all other medicines which were being taken were discontinued. Dosage was 100 mg DPH t.i.d. The trial was for one month. Assessment of subjective and objective results were verified by all participating physicians.

While on DPH, of the total of twenty-seven patients, subjective relief was impressive in twenty-five. These patients found complete or at least partial relief. Fifteen patients showed improved ventilation tests. The group of patients as a whole were generally more relaxed and, although some wheezing persisted in twelve patients, the distress was less evident.

The results of this study led the authors to suggest that DPH would seem to be a useful anti-asthmatic agent.[1]

[1]A number of people with emphysema have reported to the Dreyfus Medical Foundation that since taking DPH for other reasons they had experienced improvement in their breathing. There does not appear to be published work on the use of DPH for emphysema, but it would seem an area for research, particularly in view of DPH's reported anti-anoxic effects. (See Anti-anoxic Effects of DPH, p. 66.)

WINTER, *International Surgery* (1972),[1692] presents a detailed study of surgical techniques in bi-

lateral carotid body resection for asthma and emphysema.

In this study the author says that severe respiratory problems require careful preoperative and postoperative medical treatment. He states that in patients with severe respiratory problems he does not use narcotics and that, in his opinion, they should never be used in such cases. He further says that barbiturates should also be avoided, except in small doses, and that tranquilizers should only be used in small doses.

The author states that he has found DPH of considerable value in severe respiratory problems, both preoperatively and postoperatively. He notes that DPH appears to have special value in patients with bronchospastic problems.[1]

[1]See Anti-anoxic Effects of DPH, p. 66.

HYPERTHYROIDISM

ROMERO, MARANON and BOBILLO, *Revista Iberica de Endocrinologia* (1970),[1479] review in detail a variety of therapeutic approaches in the treatment of hyperthyroidism. They state that in addition to well-known general measures of rest, healthful diet, food supplements and avoidance of stressful situations, therapeutic measures that are commonly employed are thyroidostatic treatment, surgical resection and radioisotopic treatment. Although each of these methods has therapeutic usefulness, they are not without complications and side effects, and there is no general agreement that any is thoroughly satisfactory.

The authors state that about twenty years ago they started using diphenylhydantoin, 50 mg t.i.d., usually in combination with hydrazides, 50 mg q.i.d. The treatment consisted of alternating DPH one week with hydrazides the next week. Based on this twenty years of experience with DPH in the treatment of three hundred patients with various forms of hyperthyroidism, the authors conclude that the lack of complications in this long experience has indicated that DPH is safe as well as effective.[1] The exacting regulation of dosage frequently required with other substances, to avoid hypothyroidism, has not been a problem with this regimen.

Response to this treatment has been consistently favorable, and 70% of the patients require no change in this regimen. In the other 30% of the patients, the use of DPH every day instead of every other week, and continuing hydrazides every other week, achieved a high percentage of success.

In the last two years, as a result of their eighteen years favorable clinical experience with DPH, the authors initiated a study on a detailed basis. They state that in this study one hundred patients with hyperthyroidism have been treated with DPH and hydrazides. At the time of their report, full data encompassed nineteen of these patients. Based on this data, the authors state that the clinical effects are as follows: eight showed very favorable improvement, four favorable improvement, four moderate improvement, one slight improvement, and two no improvement. Along with these improvements, marked relief of nervousness characteristic of this disorder was also observed.

The authors state that it is significant and unlike what is often observed with other thyroidostatic drugs, that neither the size of the goiter nor the exophthalmus increased in any of these patients. Further, in some of the patients, actual decrease in size of the goiter and of the exophthalmus was very evident.

The authors state that the results have been so encouraging with these nineteen patients of the study of one hundred,that they felt that this interim report should be made. However, an enlarged study of the one hundred patients seen during this two year period will follow.

[1]Hansen, Skovsted, Lauridsen, Birk, Kirkegaard and Siersbaek-Nielsen[1125] studied the effect of DPH on serum T_3 and T_4. During the course of this study it was noted that one of two patients with hyperthyroidism, on DPH for four weeks, showed considerable improvement in the clinical picture, both subjectively and objectively. There was also a decrease in thyroid hormone levels.

GLAUCOMATOUS FIELD LOSS

BECKER and PODOS, *Symposium on Ocular Therapy* (1973),[812] in earlier studies had found that diphenylhydantoin partly protected the optic nerve *in vitro* when subjected to anoxia, cyanide or ouabain. Because of these findings, the authors decided to explore the possibility that DPH might reverse some of the effects of ischemia on the optic nerve, in humans.

The authors instituted a pilot study to examine the effects of diphenylhydantoin in glaucomatous field loss. This study involved fifty patients who were given 100 mg DPH t.i.d. for two to five months. The effects on visual fields were quantitatively recorded by means of Goldmann perimetry and/or static perimetry.

When treated with DPH, only one of the fifty patients had a worsening of visual fields, twenty-nine showed no worsening, and twenty patients showed improvement in visual fields. This salutary effect in visual fields occurred despite the fact that intraocular pressures, which previously had been deleterious, persisted. In seven of the patients that showed improvement, DPH was discontinued and worsening of visual fields occurred. The authors found of considerable interest the fact that when DPH was reinstituted in five of these seven patients, improvement in visual fields again occurred.

The authors conclude that this pilot study suggests that where the blood supply is decreased, DPH may be able to protect optic nerve function. The authors state that a larger and controlled study has been initiated by them on ischemic neuropathy.[1]

[1]Ellenberger, Burde and Keltner,[1005] in a group of fifteen patients with sharp borders to their visual field defects indicating pathological interruption of nerve fibers, did not find that DPH significantly affected visual acuity. They note that the patients which they studied differed from those with glaucomatous visual field loss. They suggest that examination of the protective effect of DPH in ischemic cerebral disease would be of interest.

GLYCOGEN STORAGE DISEASE

JUBIZ and RALLISON, *Archives of Internal Medi-*

cine (1974),[1193] report on four patients with glycogen storage disease, two with debranching system deficiency, one with phosphorylase deficiency and one with glucose-6-phosphatase deficiency.

The authors state that these patients were treated with diphenylhydantoin for more than two years and there was a good response. This was evidenced by a reduction in liver size both clinically and by liver scan. Also, a reduction in hepatic glycogen content by chemical analysis and light and electron microscopy was observed. Hyperlacticacidemia improved. Some changes in blood glucose and liver function tests were also observed.

As a result of their findings, the authors state that clinical trials in larger groups of patients with different forms and severity of glycogen storage disease seem indicated.

HEALING[1]—PERIODONTAL

SAVINI, POITEVIN and POITEVIN, *Revue Francaise d'Odontostomatologie* (1972),[1504] presented a study of the use of diphenylhydantoin locally in the treatment of periodontal disease in 118 cases.

The authors examined the effect of DPH in a gingival-paste-type ointment which was applied by the patient with massage to the gingival mucosa inside and outside after normal tooth brushing, morning and evening, and left for about five minutes before rinsing.

The findings were based both on the patient's observations and by physical examination, x-rays and in forty-six cases by histological examination of the gingival biopsies.

Biopsy results showed that in thirty-one cases there was marked improvement characterized by stabilization of inflammatory lesions and appreciable healing of the connective tissue. In fourteen cases a marked healing sclerosis was observed without inflammatory elements.

In the clinical observations the following were noted: regression, and in most cases total resolution, of the painful phenomena associated with the disorder; rapid regression of spontaneous and provoked gingival bleeding; more or less rapid resolution of infectious and inflammatory phenomena; return of normal coloring to gums; improvement in the signs of dental mobility; and no periodontal restoration, although lesions were stabilized.

The authors concluded that DPH is an effective aid in the treatment of periodontal disease.

PAYEN, *Revue d'Odonto-stomatologie du Midi de la France* (1972),[1403] reported on the topical use of diphenylhydantoin, in seventy-five patients with periodontal disease.

The author noted that with gingival massage, with a diphenylhydantoin preparation, inflammatory nodules tended to diminish in volume, considerably more than would be expected based on his previous experience. He also noted that the repeated inflammatory processes, characteristic of this disorder, subsided with increased production of collagen in the healing process. The seventy-five patients were studied in two groups. In the first group of forty-six patients from private practice there were forty-five improvements with DPH. In the second group twenty-nine patients in a hospital ward there were twenty improvements with DPH.

The author concludes that local application of DPH in periodontal disease would seem to promote the disappearance of inflammatory lesions and the production of collagenous healing.

CHIKHANI, *Actualites Odonto-stomatologiques* (1972),[894] reports in a study of fifty-eight patients, the clinical and histological effects of diphenylhydantoin in daily gingival massage in periodontopathies. The author states that the study demonstrates the beneficial effect of DPH, particularly on bleeding gums and on pain; and histological find-

---

[1]For studies on the promotion of healing in animals with DPH, see basic mechanisms studies, p. 89.

ings confirmed the fibroblastic action of DPH and the healing with sclerosis which accompanied the decrease in inflammatory infiltration.

The author states that beneficial effects become manifest after forty to sixty days of treatment and suggests a minimum trial of at least six weeks should be adopted.

GOEBEL, *Journal of Oral Surgery* (1972),[1080] reported on a controlled clinical study to determine the effect of diphenylhydantoin on wound healing in extraction sockets.

As controls, one group of patients was given chlorpromazine hydrochloride, and another group was untreated. Statistically significant improvementment was observed in wound healing in patients who received DPH before and after surgery, as compared with the control groups.

SINGLE CASE REPORTS

Although the following reports are of single cases, they are carefully reported and, since they are in new fields, they are reviewed here.

NARCOLEPSY

BJERK and HORNISHER, *Electroencephalography and Clinical Neurophysiology* (1958),[835] refer to generalities in the literature that "anticonvulsants" are not effective for narcolepsy.

The authors present a case, which they consider typical narcolepsy, that showed excellent response to treatment with diphenylhydantoin. The patient, a thirty-seven-year-old female, had overpowering attacks of sleep and other typical symptoms of narcolepsy. A thorough examination, skull films, lumbar puncture and visual fields were normal, and electroencephalogram revealed a highly irregular dysrhythmic record. On 100 mg of DPH t.i.d. the patient's symptoms left her on the seventh day. The

authors state that the improvement was marked by a complete loss of symptoms. With the loss of symptoms, appetite improved and the patient said that she had never felt so well in a long time. This condition had been maintained for eight months, to the time of the present writing.

The authors point out that the role of DPH was further evidenced by the fact that when the patient stopped taking the medication the symptoms recurred.

RECURRENT FEVER

BERGER, *Postgraduate Medicine* (1966),[819] reports on an unusual case of recurrent fever, successfully treated with diphenylhydantoin.

A sixteen-year-old boy, who was first seen when he was twelve years old, began to have irregular attacks of fever at the age of eight. These attacks would appear suddenly, last from four to twenty-four hours, and disappear abruptly regardless of treatment. His temperature would rise to 102°F and stay within a degree of this reading until the attack was terminated. Headache, vertigo, weakness, irritability, and sometimes violent rages accompanied the fever.

From 1957 to 1961 the patient missed 260 days of school because of a total of 164 of these attacks of fever. These attacks also occurred during three-month vacation periods, but accurate records were not kept.

Extensive tests for possible causes of fever all proved negative. Penicillin, tetracycline and sulfadimethoxine were all tried without effect. The boy had had no signs of epilepsy. A study of his family history showed that he had a maternal uncle who had epilepsy.

Conjecturing that DPH might work, the patient was treated with 400 mg of DPH per day and the attacks stopped promptly. The dose was adjusted downward to 100 mg (25 mg q.i.d.) and with this dose (60 mg per day was found insufficient) he has been free of fever and the symptoms that accompanied it for the past four years. On four separate occasions, as an experiment, DPH was withdrawn. Each time the fever and other symptoms returned within a few days.[1]

[1]This appears to be the only published report of DPH's usefulness in the alleviation of fever, and it is an unusual case but well documented. A number of individuals who have taken DPH for other purposes have reported to the Dreyfus Medical Foundation that their "usual" attacks of "flu," "virus," etc., have been accompanied by little or no fever. Research in this area may be indicated.

RABIES

HATTWICK, WEIS, STECHSCHULTE, BAER and GREGG, *Annals of Internal Medicine* (1972),[1138] give an extensive and detailed report on their successful treatment of a six-year-old boy with clinical rabies, with complete recovery. The authors comment that this is extremely rare, and possibly the first documented case of recovery from rabies in humans.

Many conventional and other measures were used to offset this desperate condition. Special attention was given to the prevention of hypoxia, cardiac arrhythmias and seizure.[1] Approximately forty days after the infection occurred and while the boy had been in a comatose condition for several days, DPH was administered, 150 mg daily. Four days later recovery started and progressed steadily to complete recovery.[2]

[1]The role, if any, that DPH played in this recovery is not known. However, since no remedy for clinical rabies is known, this case is of interest. It is well established that DPH is effective against seizures and cardiac arrhythmias, and it is also reported to have anti-anoxic effects. Of possible relevance is the evidence that DPH has anti-toxic effects against a wide variety of substances. See Table, p. 85.

[2]See also Pollen,[1424] reporting the use of DPH in the successful treatment in a case of cat-scratch encephalitis.

EDEMA

MICK, *JAMA* (1973),[1359] reports on the case of a girl who had edema of the legs, fingers and puffiness of the face, accompanied by dizzy spells. These symptoms occurred about ten days before each menstrual cycle.

Diuretics had been tried without success. On 100 mg of DPH, twice daily, the patient became completely free of her episodic edema. Improvement in dizziness was also noted.

SAFETY AND TOXICOLOGY

Safety and Toxicology is reviewed in The Broad Range of Use of Diphenylhydantoin, pages 57, 58 and 59. Recent references on this subject are contained in the Subject Index of this book.

Five more years of extensive use add to the evidence of the first thirty-two years that DPH is a substance of wide therapeutic safety.

For recent general reviews on safety and toxicology, the reader is referred to Glaser,[1075] and Woodbury, Penry and Schmidt.[1700]

Basic Mechanisms of Action of DPH

SUMMARY

Basic mechanism studies demonstrate that DPH has a stabilizing effect on bioelectrical activity in single cells, and groups of cells. This ability to regulate bioelectrical activity has been demonstrated in brain, spinal cord, ganglia, peripheral nerve, neuromuscular junction, muscle endplate, cardiac muscle, Purkinje fibers of heart, and smooth muscle of intestine. The action of DPH is observed in vertebrates and invertebrates and is achieved whether the bioelectrical abnormality is caused by chemical or electrical means.[1]

It has been demonstrated that DPH reduces or eliminates excessive post-tetanic potentiation and repetitive after-discharge[1] and that DPH, in therapeutic doses, does not interfere with normal function. That is, it does not affect normal transmission of initial impulses and does not impair normal resting potential.[2]

There are studies that show that DPH preserves energy compounds[3] and decreases the "downhill movement" of ions characteristic of energy depletion in nerve.[4] Additional studies demonstrate that DPH has anti-anoxic properties.[5]

Separate from the studies that have established that DPH has a regulatory effect on bioelectrical activity, and on sodium and potassium transport,[6] are other studies which report that DPH has regulatory effects on insulin and glucagon secretion and blood sugar levels. Other studies report that DPH has regulatory effects on acetylcholine, on cortisol metabolism, on norepinephrine and dopamine uptake, binding and release, on calcium uptake and metabolism, on calcitonin secretion, GABA uptake and concentration, serotonin concentration, antidiuretic hormone secretion, and on oxytocin and vasopressin secretion.[7]

DPH has been reported to diminish or counteract, in animals or in man, the toxic efftcts of substances as diverse as acetylstrophanthidin, aconitine, alloxan, amitriptyline, amphetamine, bilirubin, brain mucoprotein, bulbocapnine, corticosteroids, cyanide, DDT, delphinine, deslanoside, digitalis, estradiol, gold preparations, imipramine, lithium carbonate, mephenytoin, mephobarbital, methaqualone, methylphenidate, morphine, ouabain, phenylisothiocyanate, propoxyphene, reserpine, streptozotocin, strychnine, tetrabenazine, thyroxine and trimethadione, and of radiation.[8]

Other studies demonstrate that DPH enhances healing processes in animals.[9]

[1] Ref. 11, 90, 257, 264, 270, 289, 359, 365, 458, 462, 468, 472, 580, 582, 789, 885, 953, 954, 955, 1117, 1197, 1198, 1199, 1221, 1291, 1343, 1400, 1435, 1467, 1469, 1494, 1580, 1602

[2] Ref. 90, 257, 289, 365, 458, 472, 782, 954, 955, 1197, 1198, 1291, 1400, 1467, 1469, 1494, 1602

[3] Ref. 17, 37, 483, 739, 1071

[4] Ref. 94, 293, 387, 728, 731, 782, 834, 1012, 1025, 1144, 1197, 1418, 1662, 1664

[5] Ref. 118, 164, 263, 285, 293, 717, 804, 1160, 1216, 1374, 1419, 1576, 1591

[6] Ref. 94, 96, 144, 157, 219, 285, 287, 293, 387, 480, 481, 483, 530, 618, 645, 699, 714, 717, 728, 731, 782, 800, 834, 955, 958, 1012, 1013, 1014, 1023, 1024, 1025, 1028, 1035, 1070, 1085, 1103, 1144, 1147, 1197, 1221, 1225, 1227, 1283, 1284, 1285, 1291, 1358, 1379, 1385, 1409, 1418, 1419, 1507, 1547, 1548, 1567, 1580, 1622, 1642, 1662, 1664, 1688, 1696, 1699

[7] Ref. 91, 92, 96, 172, 219, 382, 430, 454, 502, 522, 532, 763, 776, 789, 872, 885, 896, 909, 924, 964, 1015, 1021, 1062, 1092, 1103, 1105, 1108, 1109, 1128, 1131, 1154, 1157, 1220, 1222, 1240, 1256, 1269, 1272, 1274, 1282, 1327, 1351, 1355, 1368, 1404, 1406, 1417, 1454, 1480, 1495, 1509, 1567, 1583, 1627, 1642, 1644, 1678, 1679

[8] Ref. 19, 61, 62, 80, 82, 90, 99, 149, 150, 151, 153, 154, 155, 157, 158, 171, 182, 183, 187, 213, 215, 233, 248, 249, 260, 308, 310, 318, 327, 328, 377, 403, 404, 405, 407, 410, 415, 418, 425, 451, 454, 482, 483, 504, 514, 519, 530, 567, 596, 597, 625, 685, 699, 701, 714, 753, 754, 799, 800, 805, 812, 823, 860, 880, 896, 905, 914, 921, 941, 943, 944, 963, 969, 978, 991, 998, 999, 1007, 1015, 1022, 1026, 1027, 1052, 1079, 1084, 1085, 1092, 1103, 1114, 1121, 1122, 1128, 1151, 1170, 1208, 1209, 1214, 1238, 1253, 1264, 1267, 1277, 1289, 1306, 1349, 1354, 1382, 1388, 1402, 1419, 1428, 1430, 1434, 1466, 1488, 1507, 1508, 1509, 1510, 1515, 1525, 1527, 1528, 1529, 1530, 1557, 1562, 1563, 1590, 1622, 1637, 1643, 1663, 1666, 1696, 1705, 1707

[9] Ref. 171, 172, 188, 189, 335, 336, 337, 339, 343, 499, 500, 501, 502, 504, 505, 811, 1104, 1164, 1485. For studies in humans, see Ref. 25, 127, 341, 344, 669, 730, 894, 1080, 1371, 1403, 1504

Stabilization of Bioelectrical Activity

From the earliest studies to the latest, the evidence is consistent that diphenylhydantoin corrects hyperexcitability as in post-tetanic potentiation and post-tetanic after-discharge. This normalizing of hyperexcitability is achieved without impairment of normal transmission of nerve impulses and without initial single impulse being affected.

The following twenty-four studies are in chronological order (1937-1974).

PUTNAM and MERRITT, *Science* (1937),[11] *Archives of Neurology and Psychiatry* (1938),[250] and *JAMA* (1938),[557] were the first to discover that diphenylhydantoin was an effective substance when they demonstrated that it counteracted hyperexcitability electrically induced in the cat brain. Others had previously tested DPH and finding that it was not a sedative, had not investigated its properties further.

In their experiments, Putnam and Merritt electrically induced convulsions in cats. They demonstrated that DPH was much more effective in controlling these convulsions than were the bromides and phenobarbital. They also confirmed the earlier findings that DPH was not a sedative.

The authors applied their laboratory findings to clinical use and with DPH treated a group of 118 patients with chronic grand mal attacks who had not responded to treatment with bromides and phenobarbital. The results were dramatic. Fifty-eight percent of these intractable cases became free of attacks and twenty-seven percent showed marked improvement, without sedation. Although Putnam and Merritt were focusing on epilepsy at the time, they suggested that DPH might be useful for a broad range of cerebral dysrhythmias.

TOMAN, *Electroencephalography and Clinical Neurophysiology* (1949),[458] studied the effect of DPH on isolated frog sciatic nerve. The frog sciatic nerve was electrically stimulated and the action potential with and without DPH was recorded.

DPH was found to have little effect upon the membrane threshold for single shocks. However, DPH increased the membrane stability when repetitive shocks were used. The author noted that these findings might explain DPH's effectiveness in preventing abnormal spread of electrical discharge, without affecting normal function.

The author stressed the fact that the stabilization effects were achieved with low concentrations of DPH—and he noted that this stabilization was achieved without sedation. He suggested that the protective properties of DPH could have broad applicability when neurons are more sensitive than normal, such as the conditions brought on by injury or ischemia.

KOREY, *Proceedings of the Society of Experimental Biology and Medicine* (1951),[472] studied the effect of DPH on the giant axon of squid. The nerve and its ganglion were dissected and kept in a solution of artificial sea water to maintain ionic equilibrium. The nerve was then exposed to various solutions and electrical recordings were made.

When DPH was added to the 'normal' artificial sea water, no appreciable effect on the electrical activity of the giant axon was observed. When the sea water was changed by reducing calcium and magnesium, but without DPH, a hyperexcitable state of spontaneous firing occurred in the axon. When the sea water was brought back to normal by adding calcium and magnesium, it took ten to fifteen minutes to reverse the spontaneous firing. However, when DPH was added to the solution from which calcium and magnesium had been withdrawn, it took only two or three minutes to correct the excessive firing.

The author concludes that DPH does not seem to affect normal nerve function. However, in an abnormal condition of hyperexcitability, induced by withdrawal of calcium and magnesium, DPH effectively corrected this hyperexcitability. When calcium or magnesium was omitted from the solution, the squid axon became hyperirritable for a brief period and then its fibers lost their ability to fire.[1]

[1]This provides an understanding of how DPH by correcting hyperexcitability prevents the sequelae of exhaustion. See later evidence of preservation of energy compounds (Ref. 17, 37, 483, 739 and 1071) and evidence of the offsetting of "downhill movement" of ions (Ref. 387, 728, 731, 834, 1025, 1144, 1225, 1379, 1385, 1418, 1642 and 1662).

ESPLIN, *Journal of Pharmacology and Experimental Therapeutics* (1957),[90] studied the effect of DPH on post-tetanic potentiation in the spinal cord and stellate ganglion of the cat. Post-tetanic potentiation is a state of hyperexcitability of nerve in which, following unusually intense stimulation, the threshold of the nerve is lowered to subsequent stimuli, that is, the nerve fires more easily with less intense stimuli. In its most hyperexcitable state, the nerve fires spontaneously without stimulus.

The author found that DPH reduced or abolished post-tetanic potentiation. He also demonstrated that DPH counteracted post-tetanic potentiation in other experiments on the C fibers of the cat vagus nerve *in vivo*.

The author noted that DPH had no effect upon isolated single impulses measured in spinal cord transmission, and in stellate ganglion transmission.[1]

The author states that post-tetanic potentiation may be significantly concerned in all functions of the nervous system characterized by repetitive activity, and that the magnitude of its role would seem to be in direct relation to the intensity of such repetitive activity.

[1]Evidence that DPH does not alter the initial transmission of a nerve impulse, in this case a nerve impulse measured in both the stellate ganglion and in the spinal cord.

MORRELL, BRADLEY and PTASHNE, *Neurology* (1958),[257] examined the effects of DPH on the peripheral nerve in the rabbit. Conditions of hyperexcitability were induced by both chemical and electrical methods.

The authors found that DPH raised the resistance of the peripheral nerve to being made hyperexcitable by repetitive electrical stimulation. In a separate experiment they showed that when the nerve was made hyperexcitable chemically by the removal of calcium, DPH corrected this hyperexcitability.

TUTTLE and PRESTON, *Journal of Pharmacology and Experimental Therapeutics* (1963),[365] studied the influence of DPH on neural pathways in the cat. They state that, confirming previous studies, DPH was found to have no apparent effect on single-impulse transmission. The monosynaptic reflex amplitude, whether initiated by dorsal root stimulation or by peripheral nerve stimulation, was not influenced by DPH. The authors note that these findings agree with those of Esplin[90].

However, when post-tetanic potentiation was produced by increased repetitive electrical stimulation, the authors found that DPH counteracted the abnormal state.

The authors conclude that DPH does not change single-volley transmission, but that it corrects post-tetanic potentiation.

PARISI and RAINES, *Federation Proceedings* (1963),[1400] studied the effect of DPH on the soleus nerve of the cat, and on the neuromuscular transmission via this nerve. The authors noted that post-tetanic repetitive activity which originated in motor nerve terminals had already been shown to be reduced at low doses of DPH and eliminated at higher doses of DPH.

In this study the effect that DPH had on neuromuscular transmission was gauged by its effect on twitch response to repeated nerve volleys and also on the twitch response to single impulses. Repeated nerve volleys caused post-tetanic repetitive discharge of the motor nerve terminals which in turn caused a contractile post-tetanic potentiation in the muscle. The authors found that intravenous DPH abolished this abnormal muscle post-tetanic potentiation. When a normal muscle was given a single volley, DPH did not affect the normal twitch. The authors placed emphasis on this selective action of DPH which enabled it to counteract post-tetanic repetitive activity without interfering with normal transmission phenomena.

RAINES, *Pharmacologist* (1965),[468] and RAINES and STANDAERT, *Journal of Pharmacology and Experimental Therapeutics* (1967),[467] showed that DPH abolishes post-tetanic potentiation originating in the central terminals of dorsal root fibers of spinal cats.

RAINES and STANDAERT, *Journal of Pharmacology and Experimental Therapeutics* (1966),[289] found that the effect of DPH on the muscle response to indirect stimulation is a reduction of post-tetanic potentiation (PTP). They noted that this study in muscle paralleled their previous findings and the findings of others of the effect of DPH in nerve.

DPH affected both pre- and post-junctional elements of the neuromuscular junction. DPH abolished neural repetitive after-discharges originating in the nerve terminals of soleus motor axons of the cat. The suppression of these after-discharges

markedly reduced PTP of the soleus muscle. DPH modified the tetanic contraction and often facilitated increased pre-tetanic twitch strength by a direct effect on muscle.

KLEINFELD and STEIN, *Circulation* (1968),[1221] electrically stimulated both isolated canine Purkinje and ventricular fibers of the heart and studied the action potentials. They found that DPH decreased the effective refractory period of both fibers with the greater effect being in the Purkinje fibers.

SPERELAKIS and HENN, *American Journal of Physiology* (1970),[1580] studied the effect of DPH on membrane potentials of individual cells of the chick heart growing in tissue culture. This method of separating cells from their nerves has the advantage of showing the direct effect of DPH on single cells, in this case, heart cells.

DPH was found to prevent hyperexcitability caused by both strontium and electrical pulses. Although DPH was protective against these insults, it did not affect the normal function of heart cells with regard to resting potentials, nor the maximum rate of rise or duration of the action potentials (even in high concentrations such as 1.8×10^{-5} M).

JULIEN and HALPERN, *Journal of Pharmacology and Experimental Therapeutics* (1970),[1197] studied the effect of DPH on the electrical responsiveness of isolated rabbit vagus nerve after repetitive electrical stimulation. They found that DPH did not affect the compound action potential produced by a single electrical stimulation, and that conduction velocity of both the myelinated and nonmyelinated fibers were not affected by DPH. This, the authors noted, was in agreement with the findings of Brumlik and Moretti[469] and of Bigger, Bassett and Hoffman[19]. The authors noted that the effects of

DPH were in contrast to those of barbiturates which depress axonal conduction. Further, they noted that in addition to not depressing axonal impulse transmission resulting from a single stimulus, DPH shortens the duration of post-tetanic depressed excitability of C fibers.

After repetitive electrical stimulation, nonmyelinated C fibers in the vagus nerves of control animals exhibited a period of decreased excitability. DPH, 5-20 mg/kg t.i.d. intraperitoneally for five days was found to markedly shorten the recovery period. This recovery with DPH was accomplished without an accompanying depression of conduction velocity or excitability thresholds.

RIEHL and McINTYRE, *Electroencephalography and Clinical Neurophysiology* (1970),[1467] studied the effect of intravenous DPH on the electroencephalogram analyzed quantitatively in terms of the over-all ratio of frequency to voltage. The authors note that this frequency/voltage ratio of the EEG has been used previously as an index of over-all "EEG activity."

In seven of eight previously untreated epileptic patients with unilateral EEG abnormalities, DPH was observed to produce a decrease in "EEG activity" in the range of 20 to 25%. The effect was observed within 10 to 15 minutes in the pathological affected hemisphere. In the normal unaffected hemisphere of these same patients DPH had no observable effect. Similarly, in three control normal subjects no effect of DPH was observed.[1]

[1]Another example of the selective action of DPH on abnormal cells, leaving normal cells unaltered. In this case the different effect was observed in the same brain.

JULIEN and HALPERN, *Life Sciences* (1971),[1198] studied the effect of DPH on firing rates of cerebellar Purkinje cells and their relation to abnormal cortical discharge in cat brain.

Without DPH, cerebellar Purkinje cells were found under normal circumstances to have firing rates varying from 5 to 300 Hz (average 24). With DPH a sustained frequency of discharge of Purkinje cells was maintained (average 140 Hz).

Without DPH, when abnormal maximal and generalized cortical bursts were induced by penicillin foci, the Purkinje cell discharges abruptly ceased. With DPH a sustained frequency of discharge of Purkinje cells at approximately 140 Hz was maintained, and at the same time a reduction in the abnormal discharge from the cerebral cortex occurred.

The authors note that it is of interest that DPH is here seen to produce an increase in discharge of a particular group of cells, in this case the Purkinje cells of the cerebellum, which produce regulatory inhibitory effects upon abnormally discharging cortical cells. (See also Ref. 1199 and 1117)

RUTLEDGE, SOHN and SARDINAS, *Pharmacologist* (1971),[1494] studied the effect of DPH on the hyperexcitability of a cat soleus nerve-muscle preparation. They found that succinylcholine produced muscle fasciculation and twitch potentiation.

The authors note that DPH counteracted post-tetanic twitch potentiation, but did not impair normal neuromuscular transmission.

BAKER, OKAMOTO and RIKER, *Pharmacologist* (1971),[789] found that in a cat soleus nerve-muscle preparation, pretreatment with DPH counteracts the additional excitation produced by injecting acetylcholine. The authors note that DPH selectively suppresses the post-tetanic potentiation of motor nerve terminals without impairing single-impulse transmission.

LIPICKY, GILBERT and STILLMAN, *Proceedings of the National Academy of Sciences* (1972),[1291] studied the effect of DPH on the voltage-dependent currents of the squid giant axon. The authors noted that DPH does not change the resting membrane potential.

The authors found that DPH decreased the early transient 'sodium currents', with little or no effect on 'potassium currents'. The authors suggest that this observation may be relevant to DPH's anti-arrhythmic action in heart and its stabilizing effects in peripheral nerve.

RIKER, *Japanese Journal of Pharmacology* (1972),[1469] studied the effect of DPH on motor nerve terminals under conditions of normal transmission of impulses and abnormal states of post-tetanic potentiation. He states that extensive studies in his laboratory support the finding that DPH selectively counteracts the post-tetanic potentiation in motor nerve terminals, yet it does not affect normal transmission.

DEN HERTOG, *European Journal of Pharmacology* (1972),[955] studied the effect of DPH on rabbit vagus nerve which had been desheathed. The author found that DPH in both single and repeated doses did not effect normal excitability or membrane permeability. The author presented evidence that DPH might accomplish its regulation of sodium and potassium exchange in nerve by its action on the nerve sheath. The author concluded that his results were in agreement with those of Korey[472] in that DPH did not affect either the normal membrane threshold or the normal action potential of nerve.

SU and FELDMAN, *Archives of Neurology* (1973),[1602] discuss the possibility that DPH might have a direct effect on muscle membrane (endplate) as well as the already established effect on motor nerve terminal. The authors note that Raines and Standaert[289] found that DPH acted on presynaptic motor nerve terminal in abolishing post-tetanic repetitive after-discharges. Also, they note that Norris, et al.[270] suggested that DPH acted on the post-synaptic muscle membrane (endplate) *in vivo*. The authors note that both of these studies were done with extracellular recordings, and that the present study was done with intracellular recordings.

This study utilized the gracilis anticus muscle of twenty adult rats. The authors state that by using fine capillary microelectrodes they were able to repeatedly pierce the muscle endplates and thus to record miniature endplate potentials, without the resting membrane potential being interfered with. By both electrically and chemically stimulating the motor nerve terminal, the authors were able to determine that DPH had a stabilizing effect on the excitable membrane of the muscle endplate.

The authors note that in three separate tests involving fibers from three different animals the beginning of the effect of intravenous DPH was apparent within ten minutes.

The authors suggest that the stabilizing effect of DPH on the excitable membrane of the muscle endplate could be a factor in the success of DPH in the treatment of generalized myokymia and myotonia.

DELGADO, MORA and SANGUINETTI, *Personal Communication* (1973),[954] studied the effect of DPH on after-discharge in the amygdala of the brain of awake active rhesus monkeys.

Earlier work[953] had shown that certain forms of abnormal spread of electrical after-discharge could be induced in the monkey by intracerebral electrical stimulation in several areas of the brain, including the thalamus and amygdala. Electrical after-discharge was decreased dramatically in the thalamus by DPH. The strong effect of DPH upon limiting the spread of electrical after-discharge in the cerebral cortex was also noted.

In the present study, with repeated electrical

stimulation sufficiently close together, in this case ten minutes apart, repetitive after-discharge could be obtained with 100% reliability. These after-discharges are analogous to the post-tetanic potentiation and post-tetanic after-discharges described in the studies of others. Certain abnormal behavioral sequences accompanied the measurable after-discharges from the amygdala.

Intramuscular or intracerebral injection of DPH was found to completely prevent these electrical after-discharges. (See Figure, p. 12.)

The time course of action of DPH in these experiments is of interest. DPH showed some effect in reducing after-discharge fifteen to thirty minutes after injection, and produced complete abolition of after-discharges by one hour after injection.

The authors note that in all animals, no changes were recorded in the normal spontaneous electrical activity when DPH was given. However, when the abnormal state of after-discharge was induced, DPH was found to prevent this after-discharge.[1]

[1] This study demonstrates, in an awake and functioning animal, the corrective action of DPH on hyperexcitability. The time course of this effect, correction within one hour, is consistent with therapeutic effects seen in man.

CARNAY and GRUNDFEST, *Neuropharmacology* (1974),[885] studied the effects of DPH and calcium on electrical properties of the pre- and postsynaptic membranes of frog neuromuscular junction. When muscle fibres were bathed in solutions either deficient in calcium or containing germine mono-acetate, membrane instability and repetitive firing of the fibers were produced. DPH was effective in preventing this abnormal repetitive firing. DPH also enhanced the rate of postsynaptic receptor desensitization, that is normalization of endplate regions bathed in 0 mM calcium hypertonic Ringer after depolarization by carbamylcholine.

The authors concluded that DPH has a stabilizing effect similar to that of calcium on abnormal membrane states. At concentrations of 10-20 micrograms/ml. in the bathing fluid, DPH did not affect normal muscle fibers in normal media in terms of the resting potential, effective membrane resistance, threshold membrane potential, miniature endplate potential frequency and amplitude.

MATTHEWS and CONNOR, *Pharmacologist* (1974),[1343] studied the effect of DPH on post-tetanic potentiation in the brain of rats. The authors studied the effect of DPH both on single impulse transmission and on post-tetanic potentiation. Post-tetanic potentiation of the hippocampal was induced by stimulating the commissural fibers with rapid repetitive impulses (10 Hz, five seconds duration). DPH counteracted this post-tetanic potentiation without diminishing single impulse transmission.

Sodium and Potassium Transport

WOODBURY, *Journal of Pharmacology and Experimental Therapeutics* (1955),[387] demonstrated that in normal rats, DPH decreased both the total and the intracellular concentration of brain sodium and increased the rate of movement of radiosodium into and out of brain cells. The net result was that the ratio of extracellular to intracellular brain sodium was increased.

DPH also decreased intracellular sodium concentrations in skeletal and cardiac muscle, but to a lesser extent than in brain. Acutely induced low sodium in the blood was associated with an increase in intracellular brain sodium concentration and a decrease in intracellular brain potassium concentration. These changes were largely prevented by treatment with DPH.

KOCH, HIGGINS, SANDE, TIERNEY and TULIN, *Physiologist* (1962),[1225] studied the effect of DPH on the reabsorption of ions by the kidney in dogs. Sodium, potassium, chloride and bicarbonate reabsorption were all influenced by DPH. In the case of bicarbonate reabsorption the amount reabsorbed was proportional to the bicarbonate being excreted. The authors concluded that DPH appears to enhance active sodium transport in the kidney.

VAN REES, WOODBURY and NOACH, *Archives Internationales de Pharmacodynamie et de Therapie* (1969),[1642] found that in loops of intestine of intact rats DPH was shown to increase the rate of absorption of both sodium and water from the lumen of the intestine.

CRANE and SWANSON, *Neurology* (1970),[728] demonstrated the effect of DPH in preventing the loss of potassium and the gain in sodium by brain slices, which occur during repeated high frequency electrical stimulation. Repeated depolarization of neuronal membranes makes it increasingly likely that the resting balance of ions intra- and extracellularly will not be restored.

These "downhill movements" of sodium and potassium ion balance represent the failure of active transport to restore the resting balance of ions between intracellular and extracellular compartments. DPH was shown both to prevent and to reverse these shifts, and thus it tended to restore the balance toward the normal resting state.

FERTZIGER, LIUZZI and DUNHAM, *Brain Research* (1971),[1025] studied the effect of DPH on potassium transport in lobster axons using radioactive potassium. The authors observed that DPH stimulated potassium influx. They postulated that this regulatory effect on potassium transport, in addition to the well established regulation of intracellular sodium content of nerve, might relate to the stabilizing effect of DPH on hyperactive neurons.

AYALA and LIN, *Federation Proceedings* (1971),[782] studied the effect of DPH on the electrical characteristics of the isolated crayfish stretch receptor. They observed that the resting membrane potential of this preparation was essentially unchanged by DPH. However, the authors noted that the long-lasting hyperpolarization which follows a train of action potentials was absent in the presence of DPH.

ESCUETA and APPEL, *Archives of Internal Medicine* (1972),[1012] studied the effect of DPH upon the levels of sodium and potassium in isolated brain synaptosomes. Rat brain rendered hyperexcitable by electrical stimulation resulting in seizure states was found to contain a decreased level of potassium and an increased level of sodium within the synaptic terminals. The authors noted that both these changes reflected the "downhill movement" of ions in the synaptic terminals, and that these were both pathological processes.

DPH was shown to correct both of these pathological processes in membrane function.

NASELLO, MONTINI and ASTRADA, *Pharmacology* (1972),[1379] studied the effect of DPH on the rat dorsal hippocampus when electrically stimulated and when not stimulated. When the hippocampus was constantly electrically stimulated, potassium release was observed. DPH counteracted this release.

PINCUS, *Archives of Neurology* (1972),[1418] found that DPH reduced the sodium influx by 40% in stimulated nerves. Sodium influx was not found to be affected in the resting nerve. DPH had no effect on the rate of sodium efflux in either resting or stimulated lobster nerve.

The author concluded that DPH acts primarily by limiting the increase in sodium permeability which occurs during stimulation. He noted further that DPH appeared to counteract "downhill" sodium movements in stimulated nerves without affecting normal sodium movements.[1]

The author notes that these findings are in accord with his previous study[1419] in which he demonstrated that DPH does not affect the intracellular sodium concentration in normally functioning oxygenated lobster nerves, but that DPH tends to lower intracellular sodium in nerves damaged by hypoxia, or by ouabain or by cyanide.

'[1] See also Lipicky, Gilbert and Stillman.[1291]

WATSON and WOODBURY, *Chemical Modulation of Brain Function* (1973),[1664] studied the effect of DPH on sodium transport and membrane permeability of the epithelium of frog skin and toad urinary bladder preparations. The authors concluded that DPH increases net sodium transport in both cases by increasing the permeability of the outer membrane to sodium. They noted that their results are in agreement with those of Van Rees, Woodbury and Noach,[1642] which demonstrated that DPH increased the net sodium transport across the epithelial cells of the intestinal mucosa. They noted that their findings would be consistent with the action of DPH in stimulating sodium-potassium-ATPase when the sodium-potassium ratio in the system is high (greater than 25 to 1).

The authors noted that these observations on the relevance of the sodium-potassium ratio to the action of DPH on the sodium-potassium-ATPase activity, first demonstrated by Rawson and Pincus[293] and by Festoff and Appel[94] have been confirmed and extended for brain cortex by Lewin and Bleck,[1283] and by Siegel and Goodwin.[1548]

NOACH, VAN REES and DE WOLFF, *Archives Internationales de Pharmacodynamie et de Therapie* (1973),[1385] found that when sodium is lacking from the intestinal lumen DPH causes the sodium to increase in the lumen by active extrusion of sodium from the gut wall.

WOODBURY and KEMP, *Psychiatria, Neurologia, Neurochirurgia* (1971),[1696] reviewed the pharmacology and mechanisms of action of DPH, and described their new studies on the stabilizing effect of DPH on cardiac muscle and on intestinal smooth muscle.

The authors state that the predominant effect of DPH in the brain is its anti-spreading activity on abnormal discharges. "The anti-spreading effect of DPH appears to be a result of its ability to block post-tetanic potentiation, a process that is related to the known effect of DPH to stabilize membranes, particularly when they are hyperexcitable.... Electrolytes are concerned with stabilization of the membrane, a process regulated by DPH."

DPH was found in an earlier study by Woodbury[387] to prevent the increased sodium and the decreased potassium concentrations which occur in the brain of rats made hyperexcitable by depleting their extracellular fluid of sodium. DPH was also found to prevent the rise in intracellular sodium and the fall in potassium concentration of the brain that follows induction of a maximal electroshock seizure in rats. Further, the turnover of radioactive sodium in the brain was also found to be increased by DPH.

The authors referred to the previously unpublished experiments of Watson and Woodbury on the protective effect of DPH on the guinea pig heart. They found that DPH counteracted ouabain's lethal and electrolyte-disturbing effects, and that these protective effects could be recorded on the electrocardiogram.

The authors referred to the study by Van Rees, Woodbury and Noach[1642] which demonstrated that DPH increased the rate of absorption of both water and sodium from the lumen of loops of the intestine of intact rats. The authors concluded that in both excitable and nonexcitable tissues, DPH increases the transport of sodium across cell membranes.

The authors found that DPH tended to reduce towards more normal levels the amplitude of contraction of the smooth muscle of rat ileum when it had been rendered hyperexcitable by barium ions.

The authors also did experiments to determine the exact site of binding of DPH in the cell. They found that DPH had a marked affinity for the microsomal fraction of rat brain and liver.

In separate experiments in which radioactive orotic acid was given to determine its incorporation into nucleic acids of liver and brain, DPH was found to enhance the incorporation of orotic acid into the nucleic acids of both the nuclei and microsomes.

The authors also referred to their other unpublished results which indicate that DPH "makes more energy available to various functions in the body, perhaps by its effects to enhance protein synthesis."

Anti-anoxic Effects of DPH

Although this is a diverse group of studies, they are consistent in the finding that DPH has a protective effect against oxygen deprivation.
The following studies are in chronological order (1944-1973).

HOFF and YAHN, *American Journal of Physiology* (1944),[164] studied the effect of DPH upon tolerance of rats and mice to reduced atmospheric pressures. After injection of DPH, animals withstood a lower pressure than was possible for animals without DPH. Animals receiving DPH could be taken to extraordinarily low pressures and survive.

The authors propose that under conditions of severe oxygen lack, DPH prolongs normal function of nerve cells, in particular of the respiratory and cardiac centers.

For more detailed summary see page 79, Vol. I.

FORDA and MCILWAIN, *British Journal of Pharmacology* (1953),[717] electrically stimulated guinea pig brain slices at 500 and 2,000 cyc./sec., 3.5 V. At this level more oxygen per gm per hour was used. When DPH was added, this increase in the use of oxygen was reduced.

The increase in oxygen use produced by the less intense stimulation of 50 cyc./sec., 1.3 V or 2 V, was not changed by DPH.

GAYET-HALLION and BERTRAND, *Comptes Rendus des Seances de la Societe de Biologie et de Ses Filiales* (1959),[118] found that DPH prolonged respiratory activity. Rats were immersed in water at 14-15°C, with the times of immersion varying from trial to trial.

DPH given intraperitoneally three hours before the test permitted highly significant prolongation of respiratory activity. There was a marked increase in survival of the animals with DPH.

NAIMAN and WILLIAMS, *Journal of Pharmacology and Experimental Therapeutics* (1964),[263] studied the effects of DPH on anoxia. DPH prolonged the duration of respiratory activity in cats and guinea pigs subjected to nitrogen anoxia.

It also prolonged the duration of respiratory activity in decapitated guinea pig head.

For more detailed summary see page 79, Vol. I.

BASSETT, BIGGER and HOFFMAN, *The Journal of Pharmacology and Experimental Therapeutics* (1970),[804] in a study in which thirteen isolated dog hearts were used, found that DPH protected canine Purkinje fibers in heart, during hypoxia.

Background: The authors call attention to recent reports that indicate that ventricular arrhythmias are encountered in a high percentage of cases of ischemia caused by coronary artery occlusion, and that the results of numerous experiments suggest that Purkinje fibers are involved in the genesis of many ventricular arrhythmias. Hypoxia, ischemia and release of potassium and other intracellular substances could disturb cardiac rhythm by altering the sensitivity of Purkinje fibers.

The authors note that DPH has been found effective in abolishing many induced ventricular arrhythmias in dogs, including those caused by tying off the anterior descending coronary artery, and in pigs DPH has been shown to increase the number of survivors after experimentally induced myocardial ischemia and infarction. DPH has widely been found effective in abolishing many arrhythmias in man, including those following myocardial infarction.

The authors, in an earlier study using micro-electrode techniques, had found that DPH had a protective effect on the electrophysiologic properties of canine Purkinje fibers subjected to toxic conditions, namely those induced by ouabain, those induced by low temperature and those induced by excessive stretch.

Methods and Conclusions: In the present study with isolated dog hearts, the authors state that they were concerned with the effectiveness of DPH in helping cardiac tissues survive during low oxygen tension. To determine the effect of DPH, the Purkinje fiber preparation of the isolated heart was stimulated electrically at a constant rate, and the electrical responses were measured until optimal performance was established. Then hypoxia was induced by perfusion with a nitrogen-carbon dioxide mixture. This hypoxia resulted in a sharp reduction in electrical response. The authors found that DPH improved electrical response, as measured by phase zero V_{max}, induced by hypoxia. They also found that DPH improved electrical response, as measured by phase zero V_{max}, when the Purkinje fiber had already been depressed by hypoxia.

The authors observed that DPH protected the normal function of Purkinje fibers against lowered oxygen. They also noted that when the Purkinje fibers had been impaired by hypoxia, DPH transiently improved this condition.[1]

[1]For other instances of restoration of electrical activity by DPH (in brain) see Crane and Swanson,[728] and (in skeletal muscle) see Su and Feldman.[1602] In addition, see increase in level of energy compounds (Ref. 17, 37, 483, 739, 1071). These laboratory findings parallel the clinical observations that DPH tends to increase energy levels when they are below normal.

PINCUS, GROVE, MARINO and GLASER, *Presented at the International Society of Neurochemistry* (1969),[1419] observed that DPH tends to reduce the abnormal accumulation of intracellular sodium in hypoxic nerves. But in normally functioning, oxygenated nerves, DPH does not affect intracellular sodium.

DPH was also found to lessen the abnormal rise in intracellular sodium in nerves in which the sodium extrusion mechanism had been destroyed by cyanide or ouabain or both.

The authors state: "Diphenylhydantoin has been shown to have a stabilizing influence on virtually all excitable membranes. These effects have been seen in a wide variety of vertebrate and invertebrate species." (For earlier work see Pincus and Giarman[285] and Rawson and Pincus.)[293]

SPECTOR, *British Journal of Pharmacology* (1972),[1576] demonstrated that DPH reduced the rate of utilization of oxygen by a rat cerebral cortex homogenate preparation.

The homogenates were composed largely of free mitochondria and synaptosomes.

MOSS, *Bulletin of the New York Academy of Medicine* (1973),[1374] found that DPH pretreatment protects against the development of "shock lung" in dogs.

Fourteen dogs were included in the study. Six were used as controls. All fourteen dogs were subjected to the same amount of femoral arterial hemorrhage followed by reinfusion of the shed blood, and all were sacrificed one hour later.

Six dogs (the controls) were not treated with DPH. When sacrificed, all showed pulmonary edema, hemorrhage, congestion and atelectasis typical of shock lung.

Eight dogs were treated with DPH, 5 mg/kg intramuscularly, one hour prior to the hemorrhage regimen. When these eight dogs were sacrificed, none had shock lung. Their lungs appeared normal both grossly and microscopically.

The author states that DPH is known to protect brain metabolism and function under conditions of hypoxia. This study furnishes evidence that DPH provides protection against lung damage under conditions of hypoxia, as induced by a hemorrhagic trauma.

STEIN and MOSS, *Surgical Forum* (1973),[1591] in a controlled study found that pretreatment with DPH afforded statistically significant protection against "shock lung" in rats.

HONDA, PODOS and BECKER, *Investigative Ophthalmology* (1973),[1160] observed the protective effect of DPH against oxygen deprivation in the retina of rabbits as registered on one of the two major peaks of the electroretinogram.

Thirty rabbit eyes were used in the study. Techniques and methods were described in a preceding report (Honda, Podos and Becker[1159]). Based on that earlier report concentrations of DPH 10^{-4} M appeared to be in the optimal range for this preparation. High potassium media were used. Hypoxia was induced in the incubated retina by stopping the oxygen flow into the incubating chamber.

In one of the two major peaks (PII as recorded on the electroretinogram) DPH had a marked effect in protecting against hypoxia. In control retinas, oxygen deprivation for two minutes caused the PII action potential to be reduced to 20% of normal. With DPH added to the medium, PII action potential was only reduced to 60% of normal.

In the other major peak (PIII as recorded on the electroretinogram) no appreciable difference between controls and DPH-treated retinas was observed.

Preservation of Energy Compounds in Brain

WOODBURY, TIMIRAS and VERNADAKIS, *Hormones, Brain Function, and Behavior* (1957),[483] reported that DPH increased glycogen in rat brain.

BERNSOHN, POSSLEY and CUSTOD, *Pharmacologist* (1960),[17] demonstrated that DPH increased creatinine phosphate in rats. With control values of 3.30 micromoles/gm of brain, creatinine phosphate values were 1.30 micromoles/gm for chlordiazepoxide, 4.40 micromoles/gm for chlorpromazine, and 7.38 micromoles/gm for DPH.

BRODDLE and NELSON, *Federation Proceedings* (1968),[37] found that DPH (50 mg/kg) can decrease brain metabolic rate 40 to 60% as well as increase the concentrations of brain energy compounds measured, i.e., phosphocreatine, serum and brain glucose and glycogen.

HUTCHINS and ROGERS, *British Journal of Pharmacology* (1970),[739] found that a single dose of DPH intraperitoneally (20 mg/kg) increased the concentration of brain glycogen in mouse brain by 7% at 30 minutes and by 11% at 120 minutes.

GILBERT, GRAY and HEATON, *Biochemical Pharmacology* (1971),[1071] demonstrated that brain glucose levels were increased in mice who received DPH. The authors also found that DPH significantly increased the uptake of xylose by brain slices, without glucose utilization by cerebral cortex slices being appreciably changed.

The authors concluded that DPH also may stimulate glucose transport into the brain. They considered the possibility that, with DPH, the extra glucose may play a role independent of its more obvious one as a substrate in oxidative metabolism, such as a stabilization of water molecules in the cell membrane, with a consequent stabilizing effect on neuronal excitability.

Muscle Basic Mechanisms

SKELETAL MUSCLE

SU and FELDMAN, *Archives of Neurology* (1973),[1602] discuss the possibility that DPH might have a direct effect on muscle membrane (endplate) as well as the already established effect on motor nerve terminal. The authors note that Raines and Standaert[289] found that DPH acted on presynaptic motor nerve terminal in abolishing post-tetanic repetitive after-discharges.[1] Also, they note that Norris, et al.[270] suggested that DPH acted on the postsynaptic muscle membrane (endplate) *in vivo*. The authors note that both of these studies were done with extracellular recordings, and that the present study was done with intracellular recordings.

This study utilized the gracilis anticus muscle of twenty adult rats. The authors state that by using fine capillary microelectrodes they were able to repeatedly pierce the muscle endplates and thus to record miniature endplate potentials, without the resting membrane potential being interfered with. By both electrically and chemically stimulating the motor nerve terminal, the authors were able to determine that DPH had a stabilizing effect on the excitable membrane of the muscle endplate.[2]

The authors note that in three separate tests involving fibers from three different animals the beginning of the effect of intravenous DPH was apparent within ten minutes.

The authors suggest that the stabilizing effect of DPH on the excitable membrane of the muscle end plate could be a factor in the success of DPH in the treatment of generalized myokymia and myotonia.

---

[1]See also Post-tetanic Potentiation Ref. 11, 90, 250, 257, 289, 365, 458, 472, 823, 954, 1197, 1198, 1291, 1343, 1400, 1467, 1469, 1494, 1580, 1602.

[2]The authors note that DPH did not affect normal resting muscle fiber membrane potential (in agreement with Gruener and Stern[1103] and Woodbury and Kemp[1695]), but when the membrane was depolarized with high potassium solution, DPH had a definite membrane stabilizing effect.

PARISI and RAINES, *Federation Proceedings* (1963),[1400] studied the effect of DPH on the soleus nerve of the cat, and on the neuromuscular transmission via this nerve. The authors noted that post-tetanic repetitive activity which originated in motor nerve terminals had already been shown to be reduced at low doses of DPH and eliminated at higher doses of DPH.

In this study the effect that DPH had on neuromuscular transmission was gauged by its effect on twitch response to repeated nerve volleys and also on the twitch response to single impulses. Repeated nerve volleys caused post-tetanic repetitive discharge of the motor nerve terminals which in turn caused a contractile post-tetanic potentiation in the muscle. The authors found that intravenous DPH abolished this abnormal muscle post-tetanic potentiation. When a normal muscle was given a single volley, DPH did not affect the normal twitch. The authors placed emphasis on this selective action of DPH which enabled it to counteract post-tetanic repetitive activity without interfering with normal transmission phenomena.

RUTLEDGE, SOHN and SARDINAS, *Pharmacologist* (1971),[1494] studied the effect of DPH on the hyperexcitability of a cat soleus nerve muscle preparation. The authors found that succinylcholine produced muscle fasciculation and twitch potentiation. DPH was found to suppress or abolish the muscle fasciculation and twitch potentiation induced by succinylcholine.

The authors note that the doses of DPH used did not impair neuromuscular transmission but did counteract post-tetanic twitch potentiation.

RIKER, *Japanese Journal of Pharmacology* (1972),[1469] studied the effect of DPH on motor nerve terminals under conditions of both normal transmission of impulses and abnormal states of post-tetanic potentiation.

The author states that extensive studies in his laboratory support the finding that DPH selectively counteracts the post-tetanic potentiation in motor nerve terminals, yet it does not affect normal transmission.

GRUENER and STERN, *Nature, New Biology* (1972),[1103] found that DPH protects against steroid myopathy induced by dexamethasone in mice.

Myopathy was induced in twelve mice by intraperitoneal injection of dexamethasone. Then six of these mice received four injections of DPH over a period of two days and were sacrificed. None of these DPH-treated mice had myopathy as measured both histologically and by membrane action potential. In the other six mice not treated with DPH, each had myopathy. As further controls, six mice had been given DPH alone without effect on normal muscle membrane properties. (See Stern, Gruener and Amundsen,[1594] for clinical effectiveness of DPH in a patient with steroid myopathy.)

SMOOTH MUSCLE

DRUCKMAN and MOORE, *Proceedings of the Society for Experimental Biology and Medicine* (1955),[465] studied the effect of DPH on isolated rabbit intestine smooth muscle contractions. DPH was found to produce a decrease in the amplitude of contractions.

The authors state that this direct effect of DPH on smooth muscle of intestine is important to note with reference to the use of DPH in the treatment of clinical conditions of intestinal hypermotility and spasticity. The direct smooth muscle relaxing effect of DPH would be in addition to its stabilizing effect on the central nervous system in these intestinal disorders.

VAN REES, WOODBURY and NOACH, *Archives Internationales de Pharmacodynamie et de Therapie* (1969),[1642] found that small amounts of DPH increased the release of acetylcholine from parasympathetic nerve endings in the wall of the ileum and also from the intramural ganglia and thus had a stimulating effect on the contraction of the ileum. However, demonstrating DPH's selective effect, when the contraction of the ileum was made excessive by the addition of acetylcholine, DPH inhibited the excessive contractions of the ileum. Thus, a "biphasic effect" of DPH in this circumstance was referred to by the authors.[1]

[1]Another example of the two-way action of DPH in its regulatory function, this time on acetylcholine and contraction of smooth muscle of intestine. (See also the controlling effect of DPH on acetylcholine levels in brain, Agarwal and Bhargava[1] and in heart, Bose, Saifi and Sharma,[30] both discussed in Vol. I).

WOODBURY and KEMP, *Psychiatria, Neurologia, Neurochirurgia* (1971),[1696] showed that DPH tended to reduce towards more normal levels the amplitude of contraction of the smooth muscle of rat ileum when it had been rendered hyperexcitable by barium ions.

CHOU, KUIPER and HSIEH, *Gastroenterology* (1972),[899] noted that DPH has been used in the treatment of spastic colon patients. Their study was designed to see if DPH would alter the phasic motor activity and contractile state of an *in situ* segment of the ascending colon and terminal ileum of dog.

The authors found that the wall of the terminal ileum and ascending colon became more compliant following intravenous DPH regardless of whether the wall was in its resting condition or was made less compliant by neostigmine. In addition, DPH abolished or attenuated the phasic motor activities of the colon occurring spontaneously and following distension or deflation of the lumen. The phasic activity of the ileum did not appear to be affected by DPH. DPH inhibited the increased motor activity of colon induced by intravenous infusion of barium chloride.

The authors concluded that these studies indicate that DPH decreases the contractile state of both ileum and colon making them more distensible, and also decreases the phasic activity of the colon.

FERRARI and FURLANUT, *Archives Internationales de Pharmacodynamie et de Therapie* (1973),[1021] studied the effect of DPH on the mechanical and electrical activity of the isolated guinea pig ileum, and also of the isolated smooth muscle strips of guinea pig ileum. DPH was found to enhance muscular relaxation and to regulate the response of smooth muscle to acetylcholine stimulation. The authors note that these effects are consonant with the previously demonstrated stabilizing activity of DPH on excitable membranes.

VANASIN, BASS, MENDELOFF and SCHUSTER, *American Journal of Digestive Diseases* (1973),[1644] studied the direct effect of DPH on iso-lated strips of smooth muscle of colon from fourteen humans and twenty-four dogs. The authors conclude that DPH's mode of action can be directly on smooth muscle as well as on neuromuscular junction.

The effect of DPH on colon smooth muscle was studied by chemical stimulation with acetylcholine and 5-hydroxytryptamine, and also by electrical stimulation. In both conditions when compared to controls, DPH was found to significantly increase relaxation time and decrease contraction time.

Since DPH's effectiveness was not changed by adrenergic blocking agents or by ganglionic blockade, the authors suggest that the relaxing effects of DPH were exerted on post-ganglionic or non-adrenergic receptor sites.

The authors suggest that the observed effect of DPH on isolated smooth muscle of the colon suggests a basis for therapeutic use of DPH in the treatment of spastic colon syndrome.

(See also effect of DPH on smooth muscle of bronchi,[1535] on peripheral muscle (muscle end-plate)[1602] and on cortisone myopathy of skeletal muscle.)[1103, 1594]

Cardiovascular Basic Mechanisms

PROTECTION AGAINST ARRHYTHMIAS INDUCED BY A VARIETY OF AGENTS

SPERELAKIS and HENN, *American Journal of Physiology* (1970),[1580] studied the effect of DPH on membrane potentials of individual chick heart cells in tissue culture. This method of separating cells from their nerves has the advantage of showing the direct effect of DPH on single cells, in this case, heart cells.

DPH was found to prevent hyperexcitability caused by both strontium and electrical pulses. Although DPH was protective against these insults, it did not affect the normal function of heart cells with regard to resting potentials, nor the maximum rate of rise or duration of the action potentials (even in high concentrations such as 1.8×10^{-5} M).

SINGH, SINHA, RASTOGI, DUA and KOHLI, *Japanese Journal of Pharmacology* (1971),[1557] studied the antiarrhythmic effects of DPH, paramethadione and trimethadione in dogs. Arrhythmias were induced by means of aconitine, hydrocarbon-epinephrine and coronary ligation. These arrhythmias were of both central and peripheral origin, and DPH was protective against both.

In addition, the authors state that DPH was effective against all types of arrhythmias, irrespective of the nature and site of their origin, possibly because of its membrane-stabilizing properties.

CURTIS, *University of Michigan Doctoral Thesis* (1971), [927] in a study of experimental atrial fibrillation in dogs, reported that DPH was as effective as quinidine in terminating stable atrial fibrillation which followed hypertonic solution administration.

He also noted that DPH has been effective against other animal models of experimental atrial fibrillation.

The author notes that in man DPH has not often been reported effective in chronic atrial fibrillation, although paroxysmal atrial fibrillation is reported to be prevented.[1]

[1]The papers of Singh, et al. and Curtis, above, agree on the effectiveness of DPH in atrial fibrillation in animals. However, they point up that in man differences still exist in the literature on the degree of effectiveness of DPH in chronic atrial arrhythmias. Further clinical evidence should make for clarification. See also pages 39 and 42, Vol. I.

CORONARY BLOOD FLOW

GUPTA, UNAL, BASHOUR and WEBB, *Diseases of the Chest* (1967),[496] were the first to demonstrate that DPH increases coronary blood flow in dogs.

NAYLER, McINNES, SWANN, RACE, CARSON and LOWE, *American Heart Journal* (1968),[402] demonstrated, in dogs, that DPH increases the coronary blood flow and that DPH reduces myocardial oxygen consumption.

ZEFT, REMBERT, CURRY and GREENFIELD, *Cardiovascular Research* (1973),[1711] in a study examining coronary blood flow, found that in intact conscious dogs, with the heart rate uncontrolled, DPH (5 mg/kg) produced a mean increase of 61% in coronary blood flow. With the heart rate controlled by ventricular pacing, a similar dose of DPH produced a mean increase in coronary blood flow of 57%. There was no significant change in either aortic blood flow or peripheral vascular resistance.

The authors concluded that to date DPH is the only antiarrhythmic agent which has been shown to improve coronary blood flow.

ZEFT, WHALEN, RATLIFF, DAVENPORT and MCINTOSH, *The Journal of Pharmacology and Experimental Therapeutics* (1968),[392] conducted a study to evaluate the hypothesis that DPH given prophylactically would be effective in preventing death from ventricular arrhythmias resulting from experimental myocardial infarction. The left anterior descending coronary artery of forty farm pigs was gradually occluded with an Ameroid constrictor. The farm pig was chosen because the coronary artery pattern of this animal is relatively constant and similar to that of man.

Almost twice as many control animals (eleven of twenty) expired as DPH treated animals (six of twenty). Although the sample was not large enough to be conclusive, the authors state that there is an indication that DPH used prophylactically increases the chance of survival in experimental myocardial infarction in pigs.

As a result of this experiment the authors suggest that consideration should be given to the use of DPH on a regular basis as a prevention of fatalities originating from coronary artery disorders.

CEREBRAL BLOOD FLOW

BALDY-MOULINIER, *European Neurology* (1971-2),[790] found that DPH protected against the effects of cerebral ischemia. This anti-anoxic effect of DPH was demonstrated in cats in which the blood flow to the brain was stopped by clamping the aorta.

When control animals had the aorta clamped for seven minutes there was definitive electrical silence, absence of adequate cerebral blood re-flow, and increase in cerebrospinal fluid potassium level. In contrast, animals pretreated with DPH had definitive electrical recovery, steady cerebral blood flow and absence of the rise of cerebrospinal fluid potassium.

The animals treated with DPH could be revived for as long as fifteen minutes after occlusion of the aorta. The animals not treated with DPH could only be revived within seven minutes of occlusion. (Seven and fifteen are mean values.)

CONDUCTION

WAX, WEBB and ECKER, *Surgical Forum* (1969),[1668] in a study titled "Myocardium Stabilization by Diphenylhydantoin," observed the effect of DPH on the resting potential and the action potential of ventricular heart muscle of the rat.

Intracellular microelectrodes were used to measure the electrical potentials of individual ventricular muscle fibrils. With DPH the resting potential plateau phase and the recovery period were both lengthened.

The authors note that these actions of DPH would stabilize the heart and would make the heart less susceptible to early reentry from circus mechanisms or other rapid aberrant stimuli.

KLEINFELD and STEIN, *Circulation* (1968),[1221] electrically stimulated both isolated canine Purkinje and ventricular fibers and studied the action potentials. They found that DPH decreased the effective refractory period of both fibers with the greater effect being in the Purkinje fiber.

BIGGER, WEINBERG, KOVALIK, HARRIS, CRANEFIELD and HOFFMAN, *Circulation Research* (1970),[828] studied the effects of diphenylhydantoin on excitability and automaticity in the canine heart.

The authors report that DPH 1) shortened the refractory period, particularly of ventricular muscle; 2) increased the multiple response and fibrillation thresholds in atrium and ventricle; 3) had little effect on diastolic threshold; 4) slightly enhanced the conduction velocity in ventricular muscle that was stimulated either in diastole or in its relative refractory period; and 5) produced slight decreases in automaticity in the ventricular specialized conducting system *in vivo*.

Also, in reporting on clinical experience the authors state that their experience suggests that DPH differs from quinidine in its effect on fundamental electrophysiological processes in the human heart. DPH does not prolong the Q-R-S interval and shortens the Q-T interval. These observations indicate that the drug does not prolong intraventricular conduction and suggest that it shortens the refractory period.

Hypoxia in Purkinje Fibers of the Heart[1]

BASSETT, BIGGER and HOFFMAN, *The Journal of Pharmacology and Experimental Therapeutics* (1970),[804] in a study in which thirteen isolated dog hearts were used, found that DPH protected canine Purkinje fibers in heart, during hypoxia.

For more detailed summary see page 30.

Calcification (cardiac)

RETTURA, STAMFORD and SEIFTER, *Paper presented at Northeast Regional Meeting of American Chemical Society* (1973),[1454] conducted a controlled study of the effect of DPH in mice with predisposition to cardiac calcification. This calcification was enhanced by stress.

The authors found that DPH reversed the calcification process as determined grossly, microscopically and by chemical analysis. The authors suggest that this might be one mechanism by which DPH is effective in the prevention of cardiac arrhythmias.

Norepinephrine

LEW, *Proceedings of the Society of Experimental Biology and Medicine* (1975),[1282] found that DPH increased the concentration of norepinephrine in the hypothalamus, cerebellum and brainstem in a strain of naturally hypertensive rats. The author notes that a deficiency in norepinephrine in the hypothalamus has been reported to coincide with hypertension, and that certain treatments effective in reducing high blood pressure produce an increase of norepinephrine in the hypothalamus. The author also notes that as animals get older, there is a decrease of norepinephrine in the hypothalamus.

Since DPH was found to increase the concentration of norepinephrine in the hypothalamus, the author suggests that further study is indicated to see if DPH might be useful against hypertension.

Protection Against Digitalis Toxicity

GOLDSTEIN, PENZOTTI, KUEHL, PRINDLE, HALL, TITUS and EPSTEIN, *Circulation Research* (1973),[1085] state that the efficacy of DPH in treating digoxin toxicity is well established. In reporting the results of an extensive study of isolated dog heart, the authors state that DPH, when added to digoxin enhances the inotropic benefits of digoxin.

The authors found that before digoxin toxic levels are reached, DPH ultimately produces greater increase in contractile force, greater potassium efflux and greater inhibition of sodium-potassium-ATPase activity. The authors suggest that these are mechanisms which enable DPH to enhance the inotropic benefits of digoxin.[1]

[1]Although it is well established that DPH does not impair the inotropic benefits of the glycosides, this appears to be the first paper to suggest that it may actually enhance the inotropic benefits of digoxin.

HANSEN and WAGENER, *Zeitschrift fur Kardiologie und Angiologie* (1974),[1122] by using both isolated atrium and barbiturate-damaged heartlung preparations of guinea pigs, showed that the toxic

[1]For other demonstrations of DPH's usefulness in hypoxia, see Anti-anoxic Effects of DPH, p. 66.

arrhythmic side effects of digoxin are prevented by DPH, without affecting its inotropic benefits. By the addition of DPH, glycoside dosages can be beneficially increased.

The authors conclude that DPH offers new aspects for the treatment of cardiac failure.

SCHERLAG, HELFANT, RICCIUTTI and DAMATO, *American Journal of Physiology* (1968),[1507] demonstrated in dogs that DPH consistently converted digitalis-induced ventricular tachycardia to sinus rhythm with a corresponding reversal of the digitalis-induced potassium efflux.

At the same time that the toxicity of digitalis was markedly delayed by DPH and the rate of myocardial potassium efflux slowed, the improvement in myocardial contractility with digitalis was not altered by DPH.

BASKIN, DUTTA and MARKS, *British Journal of Pharmacology* (1973),[801] in a study of the guinea pig heart, showed that DPH and potassium significantly prevent ouabain intoxication without preventing the inotropic benefits of ouabain.

WATSON and WOODBURY, *Archives Internationales de Pharmacodynamie et de Therapie* (1973),[1663] studying ouabain intoxication in guinea pigs, observed that DPH prevented ouabain-induced electrolyte changes and prevented the development of ouabain-induced arrhythmias. Under some conditions, pretreatment with DPH reduced the lethality of ouabain from 90% to 34%. The authors concluded that these results are consistent with the concept that the antiarrhythmic effect of DPH is due to an action on active transport of electrolytes across cell membranes, since the plasma potassium was normalized by DPH pretreatment.

In addition, the authors measured the intracellular concentration of sodium, potassium and chloride in cardiac muscle and again observed a normalizing effect of DPH pretreatment.

Other Regulatory Effects of DPH

Additional regulatory effects of DPH are reported in the following studies. They include the regulatory effect of DPH on calcium metabolism and calcitonin secretion, norepinephrine uptake, binding and release, acetylcholine concentration and effect, GABA uptake and concentration, adrenocortical function, oxytocin secretion, antidiuretic hormone secretion, and carbohydrate metabolism.

CALCIUM METABOLISM AND CALCITONIN SECRETION

PINCUS and LEE, *Archives of Neurology* (1973),[1417] found that when DPH was added to rat brain slices the uptake of calcium was decreased and there was a decrease in the release of norepinephrine from the cells. The authors state that it has been demonstrated that in the absence of calcium the electrical stimulation of brain slices does not result in norepinephrine being released from the cell. They also note that when calcium concentration is reduced, norepinephrine release from the cells is also reduced. The present study shows that when DPH decreased calcium uptake into the cells there was a decrease in norepinephrine release from the cells.

The authors note that the effects of DPH upon calcium uptake may be relevant to the regulatory action of DPH in other situations, including the secretion of insulin, and the contractile mechanisms in skeletal and cardiac muscle.

(See also Carnay and Grundfest,[885] p. 62.)

SOHN and FERRENDELLI, *Neurology* (1973),[1567] studied the effect of DPH on calcium uptake by synaptosomes isolated from rat brain. At low concentrations of DPH, 0.2mM or greater, DPH consistently inhibited calcium uptake by synaptosomes which had been depolarized with potassium. In synaptosomes not depolarized, low concentrations of DPH had no significant effect on calcium uptake, but much higher concentrations of DPH, 0.4 mM or greater, had some inhibitory effect on calcium uptake.

These results support the concept that one pharmacological action of DPH is inhibition of calcium transport into stimulated neuronal tissue. The authors suggest that this may be a mechanism by which DPH inhibits neurotransmitter release and in turn suppresses post-tetanic potentiation.

PENTO, GLICK and KAGAN, *Endocrinology* (1973),[1406] state that DPH, which has been used therapeutically for more than thirty years, exhibits a wide spectrum of therapeutic effects which appear to be associated with the stabilizing influence of DPH on excitatory tissues.

The present study demonstrates the effect of DPH on calcitonin secretion in the pig. Normal basal levels of calcitonin secretion were not significantly changed by DPH. When extra calcitonin secretion was stimulated by means of glucagon or calcium administration, DPH tended to reduce the level of elevation in plasma calcitonin produced by these two stimuli.

The authors state that these findings are in accord with other demonstrations that DPH does not alter normal basal function of the pituitary-adrenal hormones, or normal basal function of insulin secretion; but that when unusual stimuli are present DPH exerts a regulatory influence.

RETTURA, STAMFORD and SEIFTER, *Paper presented at Northeast Regional Meeting of the American Chemical Society* (1973),[1454] conducted a controlled study of the effect of DPH in a strain of mice with predisposition to cardiac calcification. This calcification was enhanced by stress.

The authors found that DPH reversed the calcification process as determined grossly, microscopically and by chemical analysis. The authors suggest that this might be one mechanism by which DPH is effective in the prevention of cardiac arrhythmias.

HARRIS, JENKINS and WILLS, *British Journal of Pharmacology* (1974),[1131] found that when calcium release from bone cells growing in tissue culture was induced by the addition of parathyroid hormone, DPH significantly inhibited this release.

NOREPINEPHRINE UPTAKE, BINDING AND RELEASE

HADFIELD, *Archives of Neurology* (1972),[1109] studied the effect of DPH on the uptake and binding of the catecholamines, norepinephrine and dopamine, in rat brain synaptosomes and in brain slices. Different effects of DPH were observed depending on whether the preparations were anoxic or well oxygenated. In anoxic preparations DPH stimulated the uptake of norepinephrine intracellularly in synaptosomes, whereas in oxygenated preparations DPH reduced the uptake of norepinephrine in synaptosomes. The author notes that these different effects of DPH, depending on the state of oxygenation of the nerve tissue, are in

agreement with the observations of Pincus, et al.[699] DPH was also found to regulate the uptake of labeled dopamine in brain slices.

In separate experiments the author demonstrated that radioactive DPH was bound to nuclei and microsomes, and to a lesser extent to synaptosomes, mitochondria and myelin fractions.

The author suggests that these direct demonstrations of a regulatory effect of DPH on uptake and binding of catecholamines in brain may be relevant to an understanding of DPH's effect in controlling hyperexcitability in brain produced by a variety of electrolyte changes and anoxia.

HADFIELD and BOYKIN, *Research Communication on Chemistry, Pathology and Pharmacology* (1974),[1108] studied the effect of DPH, administered orally and intraperitoneally to rats, on the norepinephrine uptake by the brain synaptosomes isolated from these rats.

The authors observed that DPH stimulated the uptake of norepinephrine when the media were well oxygenated. They note that these *in vivo* results are confirmatory of their earlier *in vitro* results in which DPH was added directly to the isolated synaptosomes.[1109]

The authors conclude that this provides further evidence for the regulatory effect of DPH on uptake, storage and release of neurotransmitters in brain.

PINCUS and LEE, *Archives of Neurology* (1973),[1417] found that DPH limits the release of norepinephrine from the cells in rat brain slices.

For more detailed summary see p. 77.

LEW, *Proceedings of the Society of Experimental Biology and Medicine* (1975),[1282] found that DPH increased the concentration of norepinephrine in the hypothalamus, cerebellum and brain stem in a strain of naturally hypertensive rats.

The author notes that a deficiency of norepinephrine in the hypothalamus has been reported to coincide with hypertension.

For more detailed summary see p. 75.

Acetylcholine
Concentration and Effect

Van Rees, Woodbury and Noach, *Archives Internationales de Pharmacodynamie et de Therapie* (1969),[1642] found that small amounts of DPH increased the release of acetylcholine from parasympathetic nerve endings in the wall of the ileum and also from the intramural ganglia and thus had a stimulating effect on the contraction of the ileum. However, when the contraction of the ileum was made excessive by the addition of acetylcholine, DPH inhibited the excessive contractions of the ileum. Thus, a "biphasic effect" of DPH in this circumstance was referred to by the authors. (See the effect of DPH on acetylcholine levels in brain, Agarwal and Bhargava[1] and in heart, Bose, Saifi and Sharma,[30] page 81, Vol. I.)

Baker, Okamoto and Riker, *The Pharmacologist* (1971),[789] found that in a cat soleus nerve-muscle preparation, pretreatment with DPH counteracts the additional excitation produced by injecting acetylcholine. The authors note that DPH selectively suppresses the post-tetanic potentiation of motor nerve terminals without impairing single-impulse transmission. (See also Rutledge, Sohn and Sardinas.)[1494]

Vanasin, Bass, Mendeloff and Schuster, *American Journal of Digestive Diseases* (1973),[1644] studied the direct effect of DPH on isolated strips of smooth muscle of colon from fourteen humans and twenty-four dogs. The authors concluded that DPH's mode of action can be directly on smooth muscle as well as on neuromuscular junction.

The effect of DPH on colon smooth muscle was studied by chemical stimulation with acetylcholine and 5-hydroxytryptamine, and also by electrical stimulation. In both conditions when compared to controls, DPH was found to significantly increase relaxation time and decrease contraction time.

Since DPH's effectiveness was not changed by adrenergic blocking agents or by ganglionic blockade, the authors suggest that the relaxing effects of DPH were exerted on post-ganglionic or non-adrenergic receptor sites.

The authors suggest that the observed effect of DPH on isolated smooth muscle of the colon suggests a basis for therapeutic use of DPH in the treatment of spastic colon syndrome.

(See also effect of DPH on smooth muscle of bronchi,[1535] on peripheral muscle (muscle end plate)[1602] and on cortisone myopathy of skeletal muscle.)[1103, 1594]

Ferrari and Furlanut, *Archives Internationales de Pharmacodynamie et de Therapie* (1973),[1021] studied the effect of DPH on the mechanical and electrical activity of the isolated guinea pig ileum, and also of the isolated smooth muscle strips of guinea pig ileum.

DPH was found to enhance muscular relaxation and to regulate the response of smooth muscle to acetylcholine stimulation. The authors note that these effects are consonant with the previously demonstrated stabilizing activity of DPH on all excitable membranes.

GABA Uptake and Concentration

Saad, El Masry and Scott, *Communications in Behavioral Biology* (1972),[1495] studied the effect of DPH (in mice) on the GABA content of normal cerebral hemispheres, and of cerebral hemispheres depleted of GABA. DPH was found to increase normal cerebral hemisphere GABA, and also to increase cerebral hemisphere concentrations of GABA previously reduced by isoniazid.

(See also studies indicating DPH enhances the conversion of glutamic acid to glutamine and GABA in brain,[532] increases brain GABA in several species,[522] and increases uptake of radioactive GABA by brain.)[454]

ADRENOCORTICAL FUNCTION

GRUENER and STERN, *Nature, New Biology* (1972),[1103] found that DPH protects against steroid myopathy induced by dexamethasone in mice.

Myopathy was induced in twelve mice by intraperitoneal injection of dexamethasone. Then six of these mice received four injections of DPH over a period of two days and were sacrificed. None of these DPH-treated mice had myopathy as measured both histologically and by membrane action potential. In the other six mice not treated with DPH, each had myopathy. As further controls, six mice had been given DPH alone without effect on normal muscle membrane properties. (See Stern, Gruener and Amundsen,[1594] for clinical effectiveness of DPH in a patient with steroid myopathy.)

DILL, *Anatomical Record* (1964),[964] studied the effect of DPH on the corticosterone response in surgically-stressed rats. DPH did not affect the normal rise in plasma corticosterone in response to the stress of a standard laparotomy. DPH was found to not affect the normal plasma corticosterone levels in non-stressed rats.

HOLDAWAY, *Proceedings of the Indiana Academy of Science* (1968),[1157] found that chronic administration of DPH to rats produced no change in weight of the adrenal glands when compared to the normal.

KUNTZMAN and SOUTHREN, *Advances in Biochemical Psychopharmacology* (1969),[1240] demonstrated that the metabolism of cortisol in liver microsomes of guinea pigs was increased by pretreatment of the animals with DPH. The authors conclude that these results are in agreement with previous observations that DPH increases the metabolism of cortisol.

CHOI, THRASHER, WERK, SHOLITON and OLINGER, *Journal of Pharmacology and Experimental Therapeutics* (1971),[896] studied the effect of DPH on the metabolism of injected cortisol in man. DPH was found to increase the turnover kinetics of this labelled cortisol. DPH was not found to affect normal plasma cortisol binding.

WERK, THRASHER, SHOLITON, OLINGER and CHOI, *Clinical Pharmacology and Therapeutics* (1971),[1679] studied, for up to twenty-four months, the cortisol production and metabolism in twenty-one patients with convulsive disorders, with and without DPH therapy. Cortisol metabolism was evaluated by the ratio in the urine of 6-hydroxycortisol to 17-hydroxycorticosteroids. During DPH therapy there was a positive correlation between cortisol secretion rates, measured by isotope dilution method, and an increase in the ratio of 6-hydroxycortisol to 17-hydroxycoticosteroids. The cortisol secretion rate was found to increase significantly only when the ratio of the hydroxycortisol to corticosteroids increased more than 0.14.

The authors concluded that this regulatory effect of DPH on cortisol metabolism was achieved with no deleterious effects in the patients.[1]

[1]See also Choi, Thrasher, Werk, Sholiton and Olinger.[896] For further studies of the regulatory effect of DPH on adrenal cortisol function see also Christy and Hofmann,[903] Costa, Glaser and Bonnycastle,[918] Bray, Ely and Kelley,[864] Bray, Kelley, Zapata and Ely,[866] Bray, Ely, Zapata and Kelley,[865] Bonnycastle and Bradley,[520] and Dill.[964] Dill,[76, 964] demonstrated the selective effect of DPH in not inhibiting the initial elevation of plasma corticosterone in stressed rats, and the reduction in the duration of the elevation of corticosterone in chronically stressed rats. See also Ref. 997.

TYLER, WEST, JUBIZ and MEIKLE, *Transactions of the American Clinical and Climatological Association* (1970),[1627] found DPH to have a suppressing effect on the artificial stimulation of cortisone secretion in metyrapone tests. The authors found that it was necessary to approximately double the amount of metyrapone to produce the usual artificial stimulation response in patients receiving DPH.[1351]

HAQUE, THRASHER, WERK, KNOWLES and SHOLITON, *Journal of Clinical Endocrinology and Metabolism* (1972),[1128] found that DPH administration markedly increases the removal rate of dexamethasone from plasma. The authors note that the metabolism of plasma dexamethasone varies considerably among individuals. (See also Ref. 776, 1480 and 1678.)

American Pharmaceutical Association (1973).[763] The authors state that when dexamethasone is used for testing adrenocortical function in patients receiving DPH, these tests should be interpreted carefully. If this test is used in patients regularly receiving DPH, a higher dose of dexamethasone has been recommended.

In spite of this the authors state that there is no clinical evidence that DPH inhibits the therapeutic effect of dexamethasone.

HOUCK, JACOB and MAENGWYN-DAVIES, *Journal of Clinical Investigation* (1960),[172] found that DPH decreases dermal water and fat and increases collagen in rat skin. Houck and Jacob[502] showed that DPH diminished the catabolic effect of cortisol which reduces hexosamine, nitrogen and collagen fractions in the skin.

OXYTOCIN SECRETION

MITTLER and GLICK, *Abstracts of the Fourth International Congress on Endocrinology* (1972),[1368] studied the effect of DPH upon the release of oxytocin from isolated rat pituitary gland. Increase of potassium in the medium was found to increase oxytocin release. Pre-incubation with DPH reduced this stimulated release of oxytocin by 35%.

ANTIDIURETIC HORMONE SECRETION

LANDOLT, *Acta Endocrinologica* (1974),[1256] found that DPH had a definite therapeutic diuretic effect in a patient who postoperatively demonstrated an inappropriate antidiuretic hormone (vasopressin) syndrome. The author noted that this regulatory effect of DPH is remarkable in that it corrects the abnormal condition but does not affect normal water metabolism.

See also Lee, Grumer, Bronsky and Waldstein,[219] and Fichman and Bethune.[96]

GUZEK, RUSSELL and THORN, *Acta Pharmacologica et Toxicologica* (1974),[1105] note that previous studies have demonstrated that DPH is useful both in the diagnosis and in the treatment of the acute water intoxication in patients with inappropriate secretion of the antidiuretic hormone (vasopressin), but that a direct regulatory effect of DPH upon the release of vasopressin from the neurohypophysis has not previously been demonstrated.

The authors demonstrated that DPH inhibits the release of vasopressin from isolated rat neurohypophysis. The effect was observed both during release conditions and after electrical stimulation of the hypophysis.

The authors note that their observations are relevant to the other situations in which DPH has been shown to have a regulatory effect upon endocrine secretions such as insulin, glucagon and calcitonin.[1]

[1]See subject index—Carbohydrate Metabolism and Calcium Metabolism.

CARBOHYDRATE METABOLISM

STAMBAUGH and TUCKER, *Diabetes* (1974),[1583] describe the successful treatment, with diphenylhydantoin, of five patients with functional hypoglycemia previously unresponsive to dietary management.

Among the symptoms, typical of the hypoglycemic patient, were chronic anxiety, extreme lethargy, chills, frequent nausea, sensory deficits and other neurological complaints. These symptoms disappeared during DPH therapy, along with the hypoglycemia.

Clinical reversal of hypoglycemia was observed in all five cases. In addition, laboratory tests confirmed this observation in both six-hour glucose tolerance and insulin level tests, performed before and after DPH therapy.

Detailed data presented for all five patients in terms of six-hour plasma glucose tests and plasma insulin values[1] are shown in the figures on p. 11 .

As seen in these figures, DPH demonstrated a regulatory effect on both plasma insulin and plasma glucose in that it brought abnormally high plasma insulin levels down into the normal range and abnormally low plasma glucose levels up into the normal range.

[1]This demonstration of DPH's regulatory effect on plasma insulin and plasma glucose levels supports the work of Fabrykant[91,92,430] and Wilson[382] on the clinical improvement with DPH in labile diabetes. See also Ref. 733, 909, 924, 959, 1015, 1092, 1154, 1193, 1222, 1272, 1274, 1275, 1354, 1355, 1404, 1509.

LEVIN, BOOKER, SMITH and GRODSKY, *Journal of Clinical Endocrinology and Metabolism* (1970),[1269] studied the effect of DPH on insulin secretion by the isolated perfused rat pancreas. When the pancreas was perfused with glucose in the absence of DPH, insulin was secreted which could be measured by an immunoreactive method. DPH had a regulatory effect in that it was found to reduce the amount of insulin released.

KIZER, VARGAS-CORDON, BRENDEL and BRESSLER, *Journal of Clinical Investigation* (1970),[1220] studied the effect of DPH on the secretion of insulin *in vitro* by isolated islets of Langerhans and pancreatic pieces. DPH was found to reduce the release of insulin in proportion to the dose of DPH employed. The effect was found to be reversible by potassium and ouabain.

KNOPP, SHEININ and FREINKEL, *Archives of Internal Medicine* (1972),[1222] reported that DPH inhibited the "stimulated" insulin release from the islet cell tumor. They noted that their observations indicate that DPH may warrant consideration as a safe therapeutic adjunct in inoperable or poorly controlled islet cell tumors.

HOFELDT, DIPPE, LEVIN, KARAM, BLUM and FORSHAM, *Diabetes* (1974),[1154] reported on the use of DPH in three patients with surgically proven insulinomas, tested with oral and intravenous glucose.

Without DPH, all patients had fasting hypoglycemia, and blood glucose rose after carbohydrate loading.

After DPH, no patient had alteration of either fasting glucose or insulin. In addition, only one patient of the three had appreciable effects on poststimulatory insulin while taking DPH.

The authors state that DPH shows no significant effect on basal glucose or insulin values and is therefore limited in its use in insulinomas. It was useful in reducing insulin secretion after stimuli.

PELKONEN and TASKINEN, *Lancet* (1973),[1404] studied the effect of DPH on the levels of plasma-immunoreactive-insulin in two patients with surgically proven insulinomas. The authors found that hypoglycemia was not abolished but that there was a desirable lowering in the levels of plasma-immunoreactive-insulin with a concomitant increase of blood glucose to plasma-immunoreactive-insulin ratio.

COHEN, BOWER, FIDLER, JOHNSONBAUGH and SODE, *Lancet* (1973),[909] studied the effect of DPH on a patient with a benign insulinoma. The authors found that DPH effectively raised the mean fasting plasma glucose concentration and improved the immunoreactive insulin to glucose ratio. Diazoxide was also found to inhibit immunoreactive insulin from the labile pool, but it continued to allow insulin to be provided by the larger storage compartment.

The authors stated that these studies suggest that DPH has an advantage over diazoxide for the reduction of insulin release. They conclude that DPH appears to be a promising agent in the treatment of certain patients with insulinoma.

BRODOWS and CAMPBELL, *Journal of Clinical Endocrinology and Metabolism* (1974),[872] describe the successful control of refractory hypoglycemia with therapeutic doses of DPH, in a patient with a suspected functional islet cell tumor. The authors state that the adequacy of the control of the hypoglycemia by DPH was evidenced by normal overnight fasting glucose levels and the absence of hypoglycemia during total fasting up to twenty-four hours. They note that it is of interest that there was a high degree of correlation between postabsorptive glucose and serum DPH levels and also a significant lowering of basal insulin levels during DPH therapy.

Current medical management of functional islet cell tumors principally involves the use of the drugs diazoxide and streptozotocin; but both agents have significant side effects. On the other hand, the authors note that DPH has been used extensively for other purposes, with few side effects.

The authors conclude that DPH can be used at therapeutic levels to control the hypoglycemia

associated with islet cell adenomas and should be strongly considered for the management of such tumors. (See similar recommendation by Knopp, Sheinin and Freinkel.)[1222]

LEVIN, REED, CHING, DAVIS and BLUM, *Clinical Research* (1972),[1274] measured the effect of DPH on the total insulin in blood after oral glucose tolerance tests, and after intravenous arginine stimulation. The authors found that diabetics of normal weight and non-diabetics who are overweight demonstrate DPH's regulatory influence on insulin secretion more than do normals.

CUDWORTH and CUNNINGHAM, *Clinical Science and Molecular Medicine* (1974),[924] studied glucose tolerance tests, serum insulin, and growth hormone levels in healthy volunteers before and after receiving DPH, 100 mg every eight hours, for fourteen days. The response of insulin to oral glucose was reduced in different individuals by 11 to 44%. Glucose tolerance remained normal, and no changes in growth hormone levels were observed.

MADSEN, HANSEN and DECKERT, *Acta Neurologica Scandanavica* (1974),[1327] investigated intravenous glucose tolerance in eight patients before and during treatment with DPH. They found that neither glucose tolerance nor insulin secretion was affected after a glucose load. In eight patients, who had for several years been treated with DPH, the results were comparable to those found in the patients before treatment.

LEVIN, GRODSKY, HAGURA, SMITH, LICKO and FORSHAM, *Clinical Research* (1972),[1272] *and Diabetes* (1972),[1273] studied the kinetics of DPH's regulation of insulin secretion by the isolated perfused pancreas.

By comparison of the results with a computerized model of regulatory control, the authors concluded that DPH exerts its regulatory effect both in terms of the labile compartment of insulin and in terms of the provision of insulin to this compartment prior to secretion. (See also Levin, et al. Ref. 1271 and 1270.)

GERICH, CHARLES, LEVIN, FORSHAM and GRODSKY, *Journal of Clinical Endocrinology* (1972),[1062] studied the effect of DPH on glucagon secretion in the isolated perfused rat pancreas. At 25 micrograms/ml DPH markedly diminished glucagon release and had no effect on insulin release. Higher concentrations of DPH were shown earlier to reduce the release of insulin as well.[1220, 1269]

The authors note that this selective action of DPH in controlling glucagon release presumably reflects the special sensitivity to DPH of the alpha cells of the pancreas as compared with the beta cells. Since glucagon and insulin act in opposite manner in the control of blood sugar, DPH is shown in these experiments to influence the release of both hormones and consequently to have at least two potential regulatory actions on blood sugar.

The authors note the reports in the literature which indicate that DPH stabilizes poorly controlled diabetes mellitus in humans.[91,92,382,430] They conclude that the results of the present study are in accord with the observations that DPH is clinically useful.

GOSSEL and MENNEAR, *Pharmacologist* (1971),[1092] studied the effect of pretreatment with DPH on the development of alloxan diabetes in mice. DPH administered one hour prior to alloxan was found to prevent the development of alloxan diabetes. Administration of DPH after alloxan had no effect. The authors noted the work of others [1220,1269] indicating that DPH has a regulatory effect on insulin secretion by the isolated pancreas and suggested that the findings of their study are in accord with the notion that DPH binds to and exerts a selective action on these pancreatic cells. The authors conclude that DPH appeared to be protecting the pancreatic beta cell binding sites from alloxan. (See also Mennear and Gossel.)[1354]

ESPOSITO-AVELLA and MENNEAR, *Proceedings of the Society of Experimental Biology and Medicine* (1973),[1015] studied the protective effect of DPH against alloxan diabetes in mice. The authors found that both DPH administered intraperitoneally and D-glucose administered intravenously afforded complete protection against alloxan. The authors concluded that both D-glucose and DPH exerted their protective effects by binding to the pancreatic beta cell.

SCHIMMEL and GRAHAM, *Hormone and Metabolic Research* (1974),[1509] studied the protective effect of DPH on normal male rats against streptozotocin-induced diabetes. Intravenous injection of DPH, 20 mg/kg, nineteen minutes prior to or within sixty minutes after administration of streptozotocin was found to prevent the development of diabetes.

MENNEAR and GOSSEL, *Toxicology and Applied Pharmacology* (1973),[1355] studied the effect of DPH on blood glucose levels in normally fed mice. DPH was found not to alter the resting blood glucose levels. The glucose values were somewhat reduced. In mice, DPH did not interfere with the hypoglycemic effect of injected insulin, but DPH did counteract the hypoglycemic effect of tolbutamide.

Anti-toxic Effects of DPH

The toxic effects of the following substances have been reported to be diminished or counteracted by DPH. Some of these substances are poisons; others are therapeutic but can have toxic effects in overdose.

TOXIC SUBSTANCE	REFERENCE NUMBER	DPH HAS BEEN REPORTED TO HAVE PROTECTIVE EFFECTS AGAINST:
Acetylstrophanthidin	327	cardiac arrhythmias and conduction defects due to acetylstrophanthidin toxicity, in dogs and humans.
Aconitine	410, 1557	aconitine induced arrhythmias, in dogs.
Alloxan	1015, 1092, 1354	alloxan induced diabetes, in mice.
Amitriptyline	1382, 1428, 1430	cardiac arrhythmias induced by amitriptyline poisoning, in humans.
Amphetamine	99	amphetamine toxicity, in mice.
Bilirubin	1388	bilirubin toxicity in that it reduces the incidence of physiological jaundice of the newborn, in humans.
Bulbocapnine	596	bulbocapnine induced catatonia, in rats and cats.
Corticosteroids	171, 377, 425, 451, 454, 482, 483, 504, 896, 1103, 1128, 1238	toxic effects of corticosteroid excess, in animals and humans; e.g., steroid myopathy, in mice.
Cyanide	699, 812	toxic effects of cyanide on nerve, in animals.
Delphinine	410	delphinine induced arrhythmias, in dogs.
Deslanoside	308, 753, 754	deslanoside induced ectopic arrhythmias, in animals and humans.
Dicophane (DDT)	701, 823, 914, 921, 943, 944, 998, 999, 1022, 1253, 1349, 1510, 1666	DDT in that it reduces storage levels of DDT and DDE, in animals and humans.

(continued)

TOXIC SUBSTANCE	REFERENCE NUMBER	DPH HAS BEEN REPORTED TO HAVE PROTECTIVE EFFECTS AGAINST:
Digitalis	61, 62, 80, 82, 149, 150, 151, 154, 155, 157, 158, 187, 215, 233, 248, 249, 310, 318, 328, 403, 404, 405, 407, 415, 418, 519, 597, 685, 753, 880, 905, 941, 963, 969, 991, 1007, 1052, 1084, 1085, 1114, 1121, 1122, 1151, 1170, 1209, 1214, 1264, 1277, 1289, 1402, 1434, 1488, 1507, 1508, 1515, 1562, 1563, 1590, 1705, 1707	digitalis induced arrhythmias permitting more digitalis to be used before toxic effects occur; and does not interfere with inotropic benefits of digitalis; in animals and humans.
Estradiol	823	toxic effects of estradiol excess, in the quail.
Gold Preparations	1525	gold nephropathy, in rats.
Imipramine	1382, 1428	arrhythmias induced by toxic doses of imipramine, in humans.
Lithium Carbonate	1637	the symptoms of lithium toxicity, in humans.
Mephenytoin	567	the neurotoxicity of mephenytoin, in mice.
Mephobarbital	567	the neurotoxicity of mephobarbital, in mice.
Methaqualone	1529	methaqualone intoxication, in rats.
Methylphenidate	1530	the severe paralysis and mortality induced by toxic combination of methylphenidate and thyroxine, in rats.
Morphine	1026, 1027	symptoms of morphine withdrawal, in rats, and morphine induced mania, in cats.
Mucoprotein	1466	brain mucoprotein induced coma, in mice and rabbits.
Ouabain	19, 153, 158, 233, 260, 514, 530, 699, 714, 753, 754, 799, 800, 805, 812, 860, 978, 1079, 1419, 1622, 1663, 1696	ouabain induced cardiac arrhythmias, in dogs, and to counteract ouabain induced toxicity in nerve, in animals.

TOXIC SUBSTANCE	REFERENCE NUMBER	DPH HAS BEEN REPORTED TO HAVE PROTECTIVE EFFECTS AGAINST:
Phenylisothiocyanate	1528	phenylisothiocyanate toxicity in the liver, in rats.
Propoxyphene	1527	propoxyphene induced dyskinesia, in rats.
Reserpine	182, 183, 1306, 1643	reserpine induced hyperexcitability and rigidity, in rats and hypothermia, in mice.
Streptozotocin	1509	streptozotocin induced diabetes, in rats.
Strychnine	90, 625, 1208	strychnine toxicity, in rats, cats and humans.
Tetrabenazine	1306	the suppression of locomotion induced by tetrabenazine, in mice and rats.
Thyroxine	1530	the severe paralysis and mortality by the toxic combination of thyroxine and methylphenidate, in rats.
Trimethadione	567	the neurotoxicity of trimethadione, in mice.

Other Studies

BEHAVIOR

BERNSTEIN and JOHNSON, *Bulletin of Environmental Contamination and Toxicology* (1973),[823] while studying the effects of diphenylhydantoin upon estrogen metabolism in pesticide-treated quail, observed that the pesticide (DDT) caused excitability and aggressive behavior in the quail and that diphenylhydantoin reduced this excitable and aggressive behavior, without any apparent sedative effect.[1]

[1]See also study by Fink and Swinyard[99] showing that diphenylhydantoin markedly reduced amphetamine toxicity in aggregated mice, and Tedeschi, et al.[749] and Chen, et al.[419] demonstrating that diphenylhydantoin suppressed fighting behavior in mice.

FERTZIGER, LYNCH and STEIN, *Brain Research* (1974),[1026] found that DPH decreased the withdrawal syndrome in rats who had been made dependent on morphine. The authors state that abrupt withdrawal of morphine is known to increase neuronal excitability in animals as well as in man.

The typical withdrawal syndrome in the rat includes a generalized increase in motor activity, body or "wet dog" shakes, escape attempts, teeth chattering, facial tremors, diarrhea, and diffuse restlessness.

Thirty rats were injected intramuscularly with morphine. Of these thirty, two groups of ten each were also injected, twice daily, with DPH. Withdrawal symptoms were precipitated by injection of naloxone HCl. These naloxone challenges were repeated frequently over a three month period, enabling the authors to study the withdrawal episodes in the rats, with and without DPH. Observations were made blind.

The DPH treated animals contrasted sharply in some aspects of the abstinence syndrome. Hyperexcitability was remarkably reduced and significantly fewer "wet dog" or body shakes occurred in the DPH treated groups. Escape behavior was not observed in any of the DPH treated rats while it did occur in the untreated rats. Although the DPH treated animals had far less withdrawal symptoms than the untreated ones, all abstinence symptoms were not completely blocked.

FERTZIGER, STEIN and LYNCH, *Psychopharmacologia* (1974),[1027] studied the effects of DPH pretreatment on the morphine-mania response in cats.

The authors note that in the cat, morphine has been classically recognized to produce a species-specific excitant or manic response. This response includes extreme excitation and agitation, with explosive impulsivity, jumping abruptly and intermittently vocalizing. When the cats were pretreated with DPH, morphine no longer elicited these hypermanic responses.

The authors say that this study, taken together with their previous study that showed that DPH modifies withdrawal symptoms in rats, suggests that treatment with DPH may prove to be effective in reducing some of the withdrawal symptoms commonly seen in human addicts.

HOUGHTON, LATHAM and RICHENS, *European Journal of Clinical Pharmacology* (1973),[1168] examined the effect of diphenylhydantoin in six normal volunteers with regard to critical flicker fusion threshold (CFF). No significant change in CFF was observed at 200 mg, 300 mg and 400 mg of diphenylhydantoin given when CFF was tested hourly from one to seven hours after ingestion of DPH.

STEPHENS, SHAFFER and BROWN, *Journal of Clinical Pharmacology* (1974),[1593] investigated effects of DPH compared with placebo on mood and psychomotor functioning in 107 normal volunteers. A double-blind procedure with crossover was employed. Substantial doses of DPH, 100 mg t.i.d. were given for two week periods. Twenty-nine different measures of mood and psychomotor functioning were used. There was essentially no alteration in mood or psychomotor functioning as determined by the twenty-nine measures in the men and in only one of the measures, mild dysphoria, in the women. See also study by Rosenblum and Shafer,[708] which found no adverse effects on sudden withdrawal from DPH in normal volunteers.

GEHRES, RANDALL, RICCIO and VARDARIS, *Physiology and Behavior* (1973),[1058] found that DPH markedly reduced the retrograde amnesia produced by lowered body temperature in rats. In addition, electrophysiological data indicated that DPH reduced the paroxysmal electrical activity induced in the hippocampus and amygdala by the lowered body temperature.

MOURAVIEFF-LESUISSE and GIURGEA, *Archives Internationales de Pharmacodynamie et de Therapie* (1970),[1376] found that DPH shortened spinal fixation time in normal rats and also in those in which spinal fixation time had been prolonged by electroshock. The authors note that spinal fixation time reflects a form of memory consolidation process within spinal cord reflexes.

GORDON, CALLAGHAN and DOTY, *Pharmacologist* (1968),[1088] reported that DPH did not appear to affect the performance of normal young adult rats, but that DPH enhanced the learning level and stable memory of aged rats for avoidance paradigms.

DPH increased the amount of brain poly-

ribosomal protein and rapidly-labeled RNA, separated by standard sucrose density gradient ultracentrifugation.

COGNITIVE PERFORMANCE

These studies deal with essentially normal human beings. For more detailed summaries, see Thought, Mood and Behavior section, p. 16.

HAWARD, *Drugs and Cerebral Function* (1970),[1139] found DPH effective to a significant degree in improving concentration in twelve college students.

SMITH and LOWREY, *Drugs, Development and Cerebral Function* (1972),[1564] in a double-blind study, found that DPH improved cognitive performance to a significant level in twenty volunteer hospital employees.

HAWARD, *Revue de Medecine Aeronautique et Spatiale* (1973),[1140] found DPH improved performance to a significant degree in three separate groups of pilots in simulated flying and radar-fixing tasks.

SMITH and LOWREY, *Journal of the American Geriatrics Society* (1975),[1565] in a double-blind study, found improvement in cognitive functions in a group of elderly normal subjects.

HEALING

Recent studies on healing follow. For other studies on healing in animals see Ref. 171, 172, 188, 189, 335, 336, 337, 339, 343, 499, 500, 501,

502, 504, 505, 811. For studies in humans, see Ref. 25, 127, 341, 344, 669, 730, 894, 1080, 1371, 1403, 1504.

FRACTURES

GUDMUNDSON and LIDGREN, *Acta Orthopaedica Scandinavica* (1973),[1104] in a controlled study (eighty mice) found that DPH accelerates healing of fractures experimentally induced. The tensile strength of healing unstable fractures and the breaking strength of healing fractures were significantly greater in animals treated with DPH than in controls.[1] In the DPH-treated animals the fractured callus contained a larger amount of extractable collagen.

The authors noted that those results in mice are in agreement with previous findings of improved healing of fractures of the mandible of rabbits treated with DPH (Sklans, et al.)[343] They note that the organic matrix of bone is more than 90% composed of collagen and that DPH has been shown to stimulate the synthesis of collagen in various tissues (Houck, et al.[172] and Shafer, et al.)[506, 507]

The authors conclude that this higher rate of collagen synthesis may contribute to the better rate of healing of fractures with DPH.

---

[1]Whether tensile strength can be used as an index of healing is uncertain since Shafer, et al.,[337] observed an increase in tensile strength of wounds in rats with DPH, while Cheng and Staple[891] did not.

SKIN

HOUCK, CHENG and WATERS, *Antiepileptic Drugs* (1972),[1164] reported that DPH increases the amount of insoluble collagen in the connective tissue of rats. In addition, they observed an increase in another protein (insoluble, noncollagenous) which they termed scleroprotein. With this increase of scleroprotein, the authors noted

a significant reduction in the amount of triglyceride or neutral fats from the tissue.

The authors note these findings in animals are consistent with those observed of improved wound healing in both laboratory and clinical studies.

CARIES

ROVIN, SABES, EVERSOLE and GORDON, *Journal of Dental Research* (1973),[1485] studied the effect of DPH in preventing caries. The authors state that during the course of a previous study on periodontal disease in rats, there had been an attempt to produce gingival hyperplasia with DPH. Although they were unsuccessful in producing gingival hyperplasia, they noticed that the DPH treated rats did not develop caries as previous studies would have indicated they should.

As a result of this unexpected observation, the authors studied the effect of DPH on the prevention of caries in rats, using controls and dividing the rats into groups of clean environment and soiled environment (infection being a consideration in caries). Under usual experimental conditions caries do not occur except when a specific irritant is applied. In this study a ligature of the first mandibular molar was used as the irritant for inducing experimental caries. They found that DPH had a marked effect in retarding caries in these ligated animals. The effectiveness of DPH was particularly apparent for five months. By the end of ten months, it was much less effective as by this point the ligation process was highly effective in creating caries.

The authors state that a review of the literature does not reveal any previous connection between the use of DPH and the inhibition of caries. They conclude that in their experiments DPH appeared to act as a caries retarder, and it was possible that there was a significant clinical application for their findings.

OTHER

Ross, *Neurology* (1965),[1483] studied the effect of DPH on the perception of pain in monkeys. Electric shocks were given to the trigeminal ganglion. The perception of pain and the ability to react were gauged by the monkeys' performance with a lever which permitted them to reduce the intensity of the shock delivered. It was found that DPH did not alter the ability of the monkeys to react promptly.[1]

[1]This is consistent with basic mechanism studies which show that initial impulse transmission is not affected by DPH and thus the initial warning impulse of pain is not interfered with. However, post-tetanic after-discharges of pain, not the subject of this study, are counteracted by DPH. (See references on post-tetanic potentiation and relief of pain as in trigeminal neuralgia, thalamic pain, Fabry's disease and other painful disorders.)

Lotti, Torchiana and Porter, *Archives Internationales de Pharmacodynamie et de Therapie* (1973),[1306] found in mice that the suppression of movement induced by tetrabenazine, and the lowered body temperature induced by reserpine, were offset by DPH.

The authors state that these actions of DPH were unique in that twelve other substances which were tested did not provide this protection. The other substances tested were mephenytoin, ethotoin, phenobarbital, mephobarbital, primidone, methazolamide, acetazolamide, ethosuximide, phensuximide, trimethadione, paramethadione, and phenylacetylurea.

Levo, *Naunyn-Schmiedeberg's Archiv fur Pharmakologie* (1974),[1279] in a controlled study, observed that DPH reduced the incidence of lung adenomas induced by urethane in SWR mice. Fifteen mice were injected with solvent used to suspend DPH, fifteen others were untreated and fourteen were treated with DPH. The animals were sacrificed after twelve weeks.

The fifteen mice treated with solvent had a total of seventy adenomas. The fifteen mice untreated had a total of sixty-eight adenomas. The fourteen mice treated with DPH had a total of forty-one adenomas (forty-four when corrected to fifteen).

DPH Metabolism

A review of the absorption, transport, metabolism and excretion of DPH is in Vol. I, page 86. These subjects have been extensively reviewed recently by others: Ausman,[781] Gabler and Hubbard,[1044] Garrettson,[1051] Glazko,[1076] Kutt,[1247] Weber-Eggenberger and Kaufmann[1669] and Woodbury and Swinyard.[1697]

The determination of DPH concentration in serum is clearly useful in cases of overdose and in cases where there is uncertainty as to whether the patient is taking DPH. A direct relationship between clinical effectiveness and blood levels has not been established for all patients. The tissue to blood ratios are of interest because of the selective action of DPH in preferential binding in brain, established in animal studies.[1]

Clinically, authors stress the need for DPH dosage to be adjusted to the individual patient and to the condition being treated. On average smaller amounts of DPH are effective in the treatment of disorders other than epilepsy.

[1]Ref. 794, 862, 1081, 1082, 1215, 1383, 1471, 1539, 1608, 1636, 1687 and 1704.

BINDING TO CELL CONSTITUENTS

The following studies demonstrate an unusual property of DPH, its preferential binding in brain. This selectivity has been demonstrated in brain cortex, in nerve cells in preference to glia cells and within nerve cells for nuclei and microsomes in preference to other cell constituents.

RIZZO, MORSELLI and GARATTINI, *Biochemical Pharmacology* (1972),[1471] studied levels of DPH in plasma and brain of rats after short and long term administration of DPH. Plasma levels of DPH were not always found to be a reliable index of brain levels.

SHERWIN, EISEN and SOKOLOWSKI, *Presented at the Annual Meeting of the American Neurological Association and the Canadian Congress of Neurological Sciences* (1973),[1539] studied the concentration of DPH and phenobarbital in brain and in plasma in rats and in seventeen patients. In only one patient was DPH alone studied. In the rats and in the single patient studied there was an increased ratio of concentration of DPH in brain as compared to plasma of approximately 1.5 to 1. This was in contrast to the equal distribution of phenobarbital between brain and plasma.

BARLOW, FIREMARK and ROTH, *Journal of Neuropathology and Experimental Neurology* (1965),[794] studied the regional entry and accumulation of radioactive DPH in both adult and immature cat brain. Autoradiography and radioassay were used to observe the accumulation of DPH in brain from two minutes to twenty-four hours after a single intravenous injection. The authors observed that the level of DPH in adult brain exceeded DPH's concentration in plasma two to threefold, from one-half to twenty-four hours after injection. This preferential concentration in brain was not present in immature animals but became prominent at one month of age.

The authors concluded that DPH is unique when compared to other compounds, in that total brain concentration greatly exceeds the total concentration in plasma.

KEMP and WOODBURY, *Journal of Pharmacology and Experimental Therapeutics* (1971),[1215] studied the subcellular distribution of radioactive DPH in rat brain. DPH was injected into the cisterna magna of rats. It was found to readily penetrate into the cerebral cortex and to localize in the major subcellular fractions. Fifteen minutes after injection, the nuclear fraction and supernatant fluid contained the greatest quantity of radioactive DPH, and the microsomal fraction contained the least. However, by twelve hours postinjection, the microsomal fraction had retained DPH to a greater extent, approximately 38% of the total radioactivity in the cerebral cortex was found bound to microsomes. Binding of DPH to the microsomal and nuclear fractions was firm and could be released only upon alkaline hydrolysis.

The authors concluded that the microsomal fraction is the major binding site for DPH in the cerebral cortex.

WILENSKY and LOWDEN, *Epilepsy Abstracts* (1972),[1687] studied the binding of DPH to subcellular fractions of brain of rats injected with radioactive DPH. The authors noted that twelve hours after injection there was increased concentration in a heavy microsomal fraction which contains mainly small nerve endings.

When subcellular fractions from brains of uninjected rats were dialyzed against solutions containing radioactive DPH, there was a tendency for DPH to bind to fractions containing plasma membranes. The degree of binding was decreased by the presence of calcium while magnesium had no effect. When both calcium and magnesium were present together, binding of DPH was the same as when both ions were absent.

The authors concluded that DPH interacts with plasma membranes.

YANAGIHARA, *Antiepileptic Drugs* (1972),[1704] studied the distribution of radioactive DPH into neuronal and glial fractions of rat brain. He found that DPH, at least in particle-bound form, has a high affinity for nerve cells and tends to remain attached to some subcellular structures of nerve cells.

NEILSEN and COTMAN, *European Journal of Pharmacology* (1971),[1383] studied the binding of DPH to brain in the rat. The authors noted that earlier work had shown that brain appears to retain DPH more effectively than plasma and some other tissues. In addition, they cited the experimental evidence that DPH's effects are mediated by its acting on and modulating neural membrane processes.

In these experiments the binding of radioactive DPH to homogenates and subcellular fractions of rat brain was studied both *in vitro* and after *in vivo* administration. The amount of DPH bound to subcellular particles was found to be small, and selective for only certain particles. Synaptosomes bound DPH but myelin membranes did not. Extracted brain lipids exhibited less affinity for DPH than intact subcellular particles.

The authors concluded that DPH's action on membrane components of brain is achieved even at relatively low concentrations, perhaps less than 10^{-8}M. This indicated to the authors that the action of DPH may be quite specific to certain key macromolecular components in brain.[1]

[1]See also similar conclusion by Firemark, Barlow and Roth[101] reviewed in Vol. I, p. 89.

TAPPAZ and PACHECO, *Journal of Pharmacology* (1973),[1608] studied the subcellular binding of DPH by rat brain cortex slices. Binding to nuclei and microsomes was observed with lesser binding to other subcellular particulates. The authors concluded that their results were in accord with those of Woodbury and Kemp[1696] and Nielsen and Cotman.[1383]

BOYKIN, *Neurology* (1974),[862] studied the binding of radioactive DPH to brain subfractions. DPH was found to bind to nuclei and microsomes, and in each case some of the DPH bound was shown to be attached to protein. As an illustration of the selectivity of binding of DPH, it was found not to bind *in vitro* to nucleic acid fractions from yeast, mammalian transfer RNA, mammalian ribosomes, and calf thymus.

GOLDBERG and TODOROFF, *Neurology* (1972),[1082] studied the binding of DPH to subcellular fractions of mouse brain. They concluded that DPH is differentially bound to several brain subcellular constituents, that this binding is not covalent in nature, and that it does not appear to require an active biochemical process. See also Ref. 1081.

PLASMA PROTEIN AND RED CELL BINDING

The plasma protein binding properties of DPH have been studied by Loeser,[440] by Lightfoot and Christian,[1288] by Lunde, Rane, Yaffe, Lund and Sjoqvist,[1316] by Borga,[849] by Rane, Lunde and Jalling,[1442] by Ehrnebo, Agurell, Jalling and Boreus,[1000] by Conard, Haavik and Finger,[916] by Lunde,[1315] by Krasner,[1232] by Lund, Berlin and Lunde,[1314] by Krasner, Giacoia and Yaffe,[1233] by Baggot and Davis,[788] by Odar-Cederlof and Borga,[1393] and red cell binding by Hansotia and Keran.[1126]

CHEMICAL IDENTIFICATION AND DETERMINATION

Methods for the chemical determination of DPH have been reviewed by Glazko,[1077] and by Friedlander.[1039] Methods include infrared studies by Elliott and Natarajan;[1006] spectrophotometric titration and determination by Agarwal and Blake,[755] by Wallace,[1654, 1655, 1656] by Dill, Baukema, Chang and Glazko,[965] and by Thurkow, Wesseling and Meijer;[1615] utilizing benzophenone as the oxidation product of DPH, in spectrophotometric determination, as by Dill, Chucot, Chang and Glazko,[966] and Chrobok;[904] vapor-phase chromatography as utilized by Van Meter, Buckmaster and Shelley;[1639] gas liquid chromatography as utilized by O'Malley, Denckla and O'Doherty,[1389] by Erdey, Kaplar, Takacs and Dessouky,[1010] by Baylis, Fry and Marks,[810] by Kupferberg,[1241] by Evenson, Jones and Darcey,[1017] by Solow and Green,[1570] by Sampson, Harasymiv and Hensley,[1498] by Cooper, Greaves and Owen,[917] by Goudie and Burnett,[1095] by Solow, Metaxas and Summers,[1571] and by Berlin, Agurell, Borga, Lund and Sjoqvist.[821]

Methods utilizing high-speed liquid chromatography have been described by Gauchel, Gauchel and Birkofer.[1054] Thin-layer chromatography methods have been described by Vedso, Rud and Place,[1647] by Simon, Jatlow, Seligson and Seligson,[1550] and by Sabih and Sabih.[1496] A radioimmunoassay method for DPH has been described by Tigelaar, Rapport, Inman and Kupferberg.[1617] A high-speed ion exchange chromatography method has been described by Anders and Latorre.[766] Microassay of DPH in blood and brain has been described by Lee and Bass,[1262] and a method for determining DPH in saliva has been described by Bochner, Hooper, Sutherland, Eadie and Tyrer.[843]

Origin of interest of the Dreyfus Medical Foundation in DPH

The interest of the Dreyfus Medical Foundation in diphenylhydantoin started with the experience of one of the authors who had personal benefits from DPH. This experience led to the formation of the Foundation in 1963. Details have been reported at a medical meeting, and also in the lay press.[1,2]

Cooperation with and from the Federal Health Agencies

The initial objective of the Dreyfus Medical Foundation was to prove or disprove that DPH was useful other than in epilepsy. After a double-blind crossover study at the Worcester County Jail, in 1966, had produced convincing evidence of broad benefits of DPH,[3] the then Secretary of Health, Education and Welfare, John W. Gardner, was consulted. Secretary Gardner made several suggestions. One of these was to have the information communicated to physicians through a national publication. Secretary Gardner predicted such publication would yield much useful information from physicians throughout the country. The Secretary's suggestion was followed (see below).[2]

Since these first discussions with Secretary Gardner, The Department of Health, Education and Welfare and The Food and Drug Administration and members of their staffs have been apprised of the growing evidence of the broad therapeutic benefits of DPH. Secretary Finch, Secretary Richardson and Secretary Weinberger have all been interested and helpful, as have been FDA Commissioners, Dr. Charles C. Edwards and Dr. Alexander M. Schmidt.[4]

FDA approved indication for use of DPH

The only FDA approved indication for use of DPH is for epilepsy. It is a function of the FDA to respond to applications for use of a new drug or for new uses for an old drug. It has not been the function of the FDA to discover new uses for old drugs. If no application for indication of new uses has been submitted to the FDA, the absence of indication for such new uses neither implies that the FDA approves nor disapproves such uses. To the best of our knowledge, the only submission for new use of DPH has been in cardiology, presently being reviewed. (See below.)[5]

DPH now in wide use

DPH is widely used throughout the world for disorders other than epilepsy. This use is based on the extensive published works of physicians and scientists throughout the world, and on physicians' personal experiences. For an indication of the breadth of use in the United States, see independent survey by IMS America, Ltd. (formerly Lea Associates), p. 97.

[1]Dreyfus, J., "The Beneficial Effects of Diphenylhydantoin on the Nervous Systems of Nonepileptics—As Experienced and Observed in Others by a Layman," Am. Coll. Neuropsychopharmacology, 1966, Ref. 707.

[2]"Ten Thousand-to-One Payoff," LIFE, 1967, and "DPH: New Wonders from an Old Drug," Reader's Digest, 1968.

[3]Resnick, O. and Dreyfus, J., Worcester County Jail Study, 1966, Ref. 704.

[4]See exchange of letters, p. 96.

[5]Patents on DPH expired in 1963. No company has exclusive rights to sell it. It is inexpensive. One of the incentives for a drug company to apply to the FDA for approval of indication for a new use for an old drug is the exclusive right to sell it.

(continued)

Exchange of letters between former Gov. Nelson Rockefeller and former Sec. of HEW Elliot Richardson.

April 19, 1972

Dear Mr. Secretary:

It has come to my attention that a great many published reports, written over a thirty-year period by physicians and other scientists, have indicated that the substance diphenylhydantoin has a broad range of beneficial uses. Further, it is my understanding that physicians are prescribing diphenylhydantoin for many purposes other than its original indicated use, in 1938, as an anticonvulsant. In spite of the evidence of diphenylhydantoin's broad usefulness, I understand that today, in 1972, its only listed indication is that of an anticonvulsant.

I realize that the Food and Drug Administration is set up essentially to rectify errors of commission. This certainly does not fall into that category. However, I believe a public clarification of the status of diphenylhydantoin by the FDA would be most valuable, and timely.

I enclose with this letter a publication, "The Broad Range of Use of Diphenylhydantoin—Bibliography and Review," that extensively deals with this subject.

I hope you will give this your consideration.

With warm regard,

Sincerely,
/s/ Nelson A. Rockefeller

_____

June 22, 1972

Dear Governor Rockefeller:

Please forgive the delay of this response to your April 19 letter concerning the current status of the drug, diphenylhydantoin.

Conversations with health officials within the Department have revealed that diphenylhydantoin (DPH) was introduced in 1938 as the first essentially nonsedating anticonvulsant drug. The dramatic effect of DPH and its widespread acceptance in the treatment of convulsive disorders may have tended to obscure a broader range of therapeutic uses.

A review of the literature reveals that diphenylhydantoin has been reported to be useful in a wide range of disorders. Among its reported therapeutic actions are its stabilizing effect on the nervous system, its antiarrhythmic effect on certain cardiac disorders, and its therapeutic effect on emotional disorders.

The fact that such broad therapeutic effects have been reported by many independent scientists and physicians over a long period of time would seem to indicate that the therapeutic effects of diphenylhydantoin are more than that of an anticonvulsant.

The FDA encourages the submission of formal applications

which, of course, would include the necessary supporting evidence for the consideration of approval for a wider range of therapeutic uses.

Your interest in encouraging the Department to provide a public clarification of the status of diphenylhydantoin is very welcome and I hope that this information is responsive to your concerns.

With warm regard,

Sincerely,
/s/ Elliot L. Richardson

Survey of Use of Diphenylhydantoin

There follows a survey by IMS America, Ltd.[1] (year ending March, 1975) of the number of prescriptions of DPH[2] and diagnosis and desired action.

Description of Method of Data Collection – The survey by IMS America, Ltd. is a continuing study of private medical practice in the United States; the study began in 1956. Data are obtained from a representative panel of physicians who report case history information on private patients seen over a given period of time.

Fifteen hundred physicians report four times a year on a forty-eight-hour period of their practice. Each physician fills out a case record form for every private patient treated. Case histories are returned to IMS America, Ltd. for processing. The books are coded and edited by pharmacists. All information is recorded on tapes for a Honeywell 2200 computer, from which the monthly and quarterly reports are compiled.

Physician names are selected at random and include representatives of all physician specialties engaged primarily in private practice.

[1]Formerly Lea Associates.
[2]This survey is of the prescriptions for the best known trade name of DPH.

DESIRED ACTION	No. Of Prescriptions (000)		No. Of Prescriptions (000)
Anticonvulsant	3057	Stimulant	11
Prophylaxis	255	Calming Effect and Tranquilizer	11
Curb Cardiac Arrhythmia	124	Antinauseant	10
Anticoagulant	121	Uterine Sedative	9
Symptomatic	64	Antidepressant	7
Pain Relief	62	Prophylaxis and Sedative-Unspecific	6
Sedative-Unspecific	46	Antispasmodic	5
Control Heart Rate	27	Mood Elevation	5
Relieve Headache	24	Antiallergic and Anticonvulsant	4
Withdrawal Symptoms	19	Prevent Migraine	4
Analgesic	17	Control Vertigo	4
Psychotherapeutic	17	GI Antispasmodic	4
Control Dizziness	17	Antihemorrhagic	3
Antineuritic	16	Relieve Headache and Anticonvulsant	3
Reduce Tension	15	Cardiotonic	3
Relieve Migraine	12	No Reason Given	1820
Anticonvulsant and Prophylaxis	12		
Sedative Night and Promote Sleep	12	Total[1]	5827

(continued)

DIAGNOSIS	No. of Prescriptions (000)		No. of Prescriptions (000)
Diseases of CNS and Sensory Organs	2,534	Circulatory Disorders	452
Epilepsy—not otherwise specified	1,052	Disorders of Heart Rhythm	107
Grand Mal	452	Myocardial Infarct	49
Cerebral Hemorrhage	178	Arteriosclerotic Heart Disease	43
Cerebral Arteriosclerotic Congestion	177	Essential Benign Hypertension	35
Other Diseases of the Brain	176	Other Hypertensive Arteriosclerotic	
Petit Mal	99	Heart Disease	33
Trigeminal Neuralgia	89	Angina Pectoris	27
Cerebral Embolism/Thrombosis	80	Myocardial Occlusion	26
Cerebral Paralysis/Seizure	48	Coronary Artery Disease with Selected	
Stroke—not otherwise specified	38	Complications	26
Other Cerebral Paralysis	28	Arteriosclerosis without Gangrene	23
Migraine	20	Myocardial Occlusions with Complications	17
Facial Paralysis	20	Arteriosclerotic Coronary Artery Disease	17
Late Effects of Intracranial Abscess	16	Heart Block	9
Subarachnoid Hemorrhage	10		
Intracranial Spinal Abscess	10	Specific Conditions without Sickness	386
Other Neuralgia or Neuritis	9	Surgical Aftercare	361
		Medical Aftercare	25
Symptoms and Senility	1,354		
Convulsions	1,145	Neoplasms	306
Syncope or Collapse	44	Malignant Neoplasms—Other	
Encephalopathy	27	Unspecified Sites	103
Jacksonian Epilepsy	26	Unspecified Neoplasms Brain/Nervous	
Headache—not otherwise specified	22	System	60
Vertigo	13	Malignant Neoplasms of the Brain	41
Tension Headache	12	Malignant Neoplasms of the Nervous	
Other Ill Defined Conditions	12	System—Unspecified	24
		Benign Neoplasms of the Brain or	
Mental Disorders	656	Other Parts of the Nervous System	22
Unspecified Alcoholism	118	Malignant Neoplasms of the Lung—	
Chronic Alcoholism	113	Unspecified	19
Other Drug Addiction	74	Malignant Neoplasms of Thoracic Organs	15
Acute Alcoholism	45		
Depressive Reaction	44	Accidents and Poisoning	228
Other Mental Deficiency	41	Head Injuries	129
Primary Childhood Behavior Disorders	37	Other Accidents—Poisoning	35
Other Schizophrenia	24	Effects of Poisons	28
Alcoholic Psychosis	23	Injury of Nerves of Spinal Cord	21
Presenile Psychosis	21	Fractures	16
Hysteria—not otherwise specified	21		
Psychosis with Organic Brain Disorder	18	All Others	212
Neurotic Depressive Reaction	16		
Other Pathological Personality	15		
Epileptic Psychosis	13	Total[1]	6127

[1]Since occasionally more than one diagnosis is given per prescription, the total for diagnosis is not exactly the same as the total for desired action.

Combined Clinical Uses and Basic Mechanisms of Action

The descriptive terms used in this index are those of the authors of the papers.

Although effort has been made to include all pertinent references, it is to be expected that there will be errors and omissions.

Each reference number refers to a specific publication (see References, Vol. I page 117 and Vol. II page 119). Frequently a reference is listed under more than one subject.

CARDIAC *(continued)*

References

References which are summarized in the text are indicated by the page number of the summary listed to the right of the reference. See also Subject Index.

These references start at 751. The first 750 references are in Vol. I, The Broad Range of Use of DPH.

Page

751. ADAMSKA-DYNIEWSKA, H., Evaluation of myocardial contractility after hydantoinal and ouabain based polycardiographic methods, *Wiad. Lek.*, 23: 1749-1754, 1970.

752. ADAMSKA-DYNIEWSKA, H., Hydantoinal—New use of an old drug, *Wiad. Lek.*, 23: 1111-1115, 1970.

753. ADAMSKA-DYNIEWSKA, H., The effect of diphenylhydantoin sodium given with cardiac glycosides on the left ventricular systole dynamics, *Pol. Med. J.*, 9: 304-308, 1970. — *24*

754. ADAMSKA-DYNIEWSKA, H., The value of diphenylhydantoin for combating the rhythm and conduction disorders induced by cardiac glycosides, *Biul. Wojskowej. Akad. Medy.*, 14: 71-77, 1971. — *86*

755. AGARWAL, S. P. and BLAKE, M. I., Differentiating spectrophotometric titration of phenobarbital-diphenylhydantoin combinations in nonaqueous medium, *Anal. Chem.*, 41: 1104-1106, 1969.

756. ALARCON-SEGOVIA, D., FISHBEIN, E., REYES, P. A., DIES, H., and SHWADSKY, S., Antinuclear antibodies in patients on anticonvulsant therapy, *Clin. Exp. Immunol.*, 12: 39-47, 1972.

757. ALEXANDER, E., Medical management of closed head injuries, *Clin. Neurosurg.*, 19: 240-250, 1972.

758. ALEXANDER, E., Surgical management of head injuries in children in the acute phase, *Clin. Neurosurg.*, 19: 251-262, 1972.

759. ALLEN, C. D. and KLIPSTEIN, F. A., Brain folate concentration in folate-deficient rats receiving diphenylhydantoin, *Neurology*, 20: 403, 1970.

760. ALLEN, J. D., KOFI EKUE, J. M., SHANKS, R. G., and ZAIDI, S. A., The effect on experimental cardiac arrhythmias of a new anticonvulsant agent, Ko 1173 and its comparison with phenytoin and procainamide, *Brit. J. Pharmacol.*, 39: 183-184, 1970.

761. ALVAREZ, W. C., *Nerves in collision*, Pyramid House, New York, 1972. — *13*

762. AMERICAN MEDICAL ASSOCIATION COUNCIL ON DRUGS, *AMA drug evaluations*, 12-13 AMA, Chicago, 1971.

763. AMERICAN PHARMACEUTICAL ASSOCIATION, *Evaluations of drug interactions*, Washington, 1973. — *81*

764. ANDERSON, D. C., DAVIS, R. J., DOVE, J. T., and GRIGGS, R. C., Cardiac conduction during treatment of myotonia, *Neurology*, 23: 390, 1973. — *43*

765. ANDERSON, R. J. and RAINES, A., Suppression by Diphenylhydantoin of afferent discharges arising in muscle spindles of the triceps surae of the cat, *J. Pharmacol. Exp. Ther.*, 191: 290-299, 1974.

766. ANDERS, M. W. and LATORRE, J. P., High-speed ion exchange chromatography of barbiturates, diphenylhydantoin, and their hydroxylated metabolites, *Anal. Chem.*, 42: 1430-1432, 1970.

767. ANDREASEN, B., FROLAND, A., SKOVSTED, L., ANDERSEN, S. A., and HAUGE, M., Diphenylhydantoin half-life in man and its inhibition by phenylbutazone: the role of genetic factors, *Acta Med. Scand.*, 193: 561-564, 1973.

768. ANDREASEN, P. B., HANSEN, J. M., SKOVSTED, L., and SIERSBAEK-NIELSEN, K., Folic acid and the half-life of diphenylhydantoin in man, *Acta Neurol. Scand.*, 47: 117-119, 1971.

769. ANDREASEN, P. B., HANSEN, J. M., SKOVSTED, L., and SIERSBAEK-NIELSEN, K., Folic acid and phenytoin metabolism, *Epilepsy Abstracts*, 4: 221, 1971.

770. ANDREASEN, P. B., LYNGBYE, J., and TROLLE, E., Tests for abnormalities in liver function during long-term diphenylhydantoin therapy in epileptic out-patients. *Acta Med. Scand.*, 194: 261-264, 1973.

771. ARIYOSHI, T. and TAKABATAKE, E., Effect of diphenylhydantoin on the drug metabolism and the fatty acid composition of phospholipids in hepatic microsomes, *Chem. Pharm. Bull.*, 20: 180-184, 1972.

772. ARIYOSHI, T., ZANGE, M., and REMMER, H., Effects of diphenylhydantoin on the liver constituents and the microsomal drug metabolism enzyme systems in the partially hepatectomized rats, *J. Pharm. Soc. Jap.*, 94: 526-530, 1974.

773. ARKY, R. A., Diphenylhydantoin and the beta cell, *New Eng. J. Med.*, 286: 371-372, 1972.

REFERENCES

774. ARNOLD, K. and GERBER, N., The rate of decline of diphenylhydantoin in human plasma, *Clin. Pharmacol. Ther.*, 11: 121-134, 1970.

775. ARNOLD, K., GERBER, N., and LEVY, G., Absorption and dissolution studies on sodium diphenylhydantoin capsules, *Canad. J. Pharm. Sci.*, 5: 89-92, 1970.

776. ASFELDT, V. H. and BUHL, J., Inhibitory effect of diphenylhydantoin on the feedback control of corticotrophin release, *Acta Endocrinol.*, 61: 551-560, 1969.

777. ATKINSON, A. J., JR., Clinical use of blood levels of cardiac drugs, *Mod. Conc. Cardiovasc. Dis.*, 42: 1-4, 1973.

778. ATKINSON, A. J., JR., Individualization of anticonvulsant therapy, *Med. Clin. N. Amer.*, 58: 1037-1050, 1974.

779. ATKINSON, A. J., JR., MacGEE, J., STRONG, J., GARTEIZ, D., and GAFFNEY, T. E., Identification of 5-meta-hydroxyphenyl-5-phenylhydantoin as a metabolite of diphenylhydantoin, *Biochem. Pharmacol.*, 19: 2483-2491, 1970.

780. ATKINSON, A. J., Jr. and DAVISON, R., Diphenylhydantoin as an antiarrhythmic drug, *Ann. Rev. Med.*, 25: 99-113, 1974.

781. AUSMAN, J. I., New developments in anticonvulsant therapy, *Postgrad. Med.*, 48: 122-127, 1970.

782. AYALA, G. F. and LIN, S., Effect of diphenylhydantoin on an isolated neuron, *Fed. Proc.*, 30: Abstract 67, 1971. *63*

783. AZARNOFF, D. L., Clinical implications of drug metabolism—introduction, *Chem. Biol. Interactions*, 3: 241-242, 1971.

784. AZZARO, A. J. and GUTRECHT, J. A., The effect of diphenylhydantoin (DPH) on the *in vitro* accumulation and catabolism of H³-1-norepinephrine (H³-NE) in cerebral cortex slices, *Neurology*, 23: 431, 1973.

785. AZZARO, A. J., GUTRECHT, J. A., and SMITH, D. J., Effect of diphenylhydantoin on the uptake and catabolism of L-(3H) norepinephrine *in vitro* in rat cerebral cortex tissue, *Biochem. Pharmacol.*, 22: 2719-2729, 1973.

786. BABB, R. R. and ECKMAN, P. B., Abdominal epilepsy, *JAMA*, 222: 65-66, 1972.

787. BACH-Y-RITA, G., LION, J. R., CLIMENT, C. E., and ERVIN, F. R., Episodic dyscontrol: A study of 130   *16* violent patients, *Amer. J. Psychiat.*, 127: 49-54, 1971.

788. BAGGOT, J. D. and DAVIS, L. E., Comparative study of plasma protein binding of diphenylhydantoin, *Comp. Gen. Pharmacol.*, 4: 399-404, 1973.

789. BAKER, T., OKAMOTO, M., and RIKER, W. F., Diphenylhydantoin (DPH) suppression of motor nerve   *60* terminal (MNT) excitation by acetylcholine (ACh), *Pharmacologist*, 13: 265, 1971.

790. BALDY-MOULINIER, M., Cerebral blood flow and membrane ionic pump, *Europ. Neurol.*, 6: 107-113,   *32* 1971/72.

791. BALLEK, R. E., REIDENBERG, M. M., and ORR, L., Inhibition of diphenylhydantoin metabolism by chloramphenicol, *Lancet*, 150, 1973.

792. BARATIERI, A., GAGLIARDI, V., and SIMONETTI, E., Further studies on effect of diphenylhydantoin sodium on oro facial tissues in offspring of female mice, *Epilepsy Abstracts*, 6: 91, 1973.

793. BARBEDO, A. S., and BANKS, T., Paroxysmal supraventricular tachycardia, *New Eng. J. Med.*, 288: 51, 1973.

794. BARLOW, C. F., Diphenylhydantoin-2-C¹⁴ in cat brain, *J. Neuropath. Exp. Neurol.*, 22: 348-349, 1965.   *92*

795. BARO, W. Z., The non-convulsive convulsive disorder—its diagnosis and treatment, *Western Med.*, March, 1966.

796. BARSKY, P., A clinical variant of tic convulsif, *J. Pediat.*, 71: 417-419, 1967.   *19*

797. BARTTER, F. C. and SCHWARTZ, W. B., The syndrome of inappropriate secretion of antidiuretic hormone, *Amer. J. Med.*, 42: 790-806, 1967.

798. BASHOUR, F. A., COFFMAN, G. K., and ASHBY, E. A., Effect of diphenylhydantoin (Dilantin) on oxygen uptake by Sarcina lutea, *Clin. Res.*, 14: 439, 1966.

799. Baskin, S. I. and Dutta, S., Effects of antiarrhythmic drugs and ethacrynic acid on the accumulation of *86* ouabain-H by the isolated guinea pig heart, *Fed. Proc.*, 29: 739, 1970.

800. Baskin, S. I. and Dutta, S., Relationships between prevention of ouabain (O) induced arrhythmia by *86* diphenylhydantoin (DPH) and potassium (K) and their effects on ouabain accumulation and electrolyte composition in the heart, *Fed. Proc.*, 30: 394, 1971.

801. Baskin, S. I., Dutta, S., and Marks, B. H., The effects of diphenylhydantoin and potassium on the *34* biological activity of ouabain in the guinea-pig heart, *Brit. J. Pharmacol.*, 47: 85-96, 1973.

802. Baskin, S. I., Melrose, B. L., Ferguson, R. K., Akera, T., and Brody, T. M., The effect of diphenylhydantoin on ouabain-induced arrhythmia and on the formation and dissociation of the ouabain-enzyme complex, *Personal Communication*, 1973.

803. Bassett, A. L., Bigger, J. T., and Hoffman, B. F., Effect of diphenylhydantoin on cat heart muscle, *Circulation*, 35 & 36: 61, 1967.

804. Bassett, A. L., Bigger, J. T., and Hoffman, B. F., Protective action of DPH on canine Purkinje fibers *30* during hypoxia, *J. Pharmacol. Exp. Ther.*, 173: 336-343, 1970.

805. BasuRay, B. N., Dutta, S. N., and Pradhan, S. N., Central action of ouabain: effects of propranolol and *86* diphenylhydantoin on ouabain-induced arrhythmias, *Fed. Proc.*, 30: Abstract 189, 1971.

806. Baugh, C. M. and Krumdieck, C. L., Effects of phenytoin on folic-acid conjugases in man, *Lancet*, 519-522, 1969.

807. Baughmam, F. A. and Randinitis, E. J., Passage of diphenylhydantoin across the placenta, *JAMA*, 213: 466, 1970.

808. Baxter, M. G., Miller, A. A., and Webster, R. A., Some studies on the convulsant action of folic acid, *Brit. J. Pharmacol.*, 48: 350-351, 1973.

809. Baylis, E. M., Crowley, J. M., Preece, J. M., Sylvester, P. E., and Marks, V., Influence of folic acid on blood-phenytoin levels, *Lancet*, 1: 62-64, 1971.

810. Baylis, E. M., Fry, D. E., and Marks, V., Micro-determination of serum phenobarbitone and diphenylhydantoin by gas-liquid chromatography, *Clin. Chim. Acta*, 30: 93-103, 1970.

811. Bazin, S. and Delaunay, A., Effect of phenytoin on the maturation of collagen in normal skin and granulomatous tissue, *C. R. Acad. Sci. Ser. D.*, 275: 509-511, 1972.

812. Becker, B. and Podos, S. M., Diphenylhydantoin and its use in optic nerve disease, *Symposium on* *50* *Ocular Therapy*, Vol. VI, I. H. Leopold, Ed., C. V. Mosby Co., St. Louis, 1973.

813. Becker, B., Stamper, R. L., Asseff, C., and Podos, S. M., Effect of diphenylhydantoin on glaucomatous field loss, *Trans. Amer. Acad. Opthal. Otolaryng.*, 76: 412-422, 1972.

814. Beernink, D. H. and Miller, J. J., Anticonvulsant induced antinuclear antibodies and lupus like disease in children, *Epilepsy Abstracts*, 6: 210, 1973.

815. Bell, W. E. and McCormick, W. F., Striatopallidonigral degeneration, *Arch. Dis. Child.*, 46: 533-538, 1971.

816. Benaim, R., Chapelle, M., and Chiche, P., Action of diphenylhydantoin on atrioventricular and intra- *26* ventricular conduction in humans, *Ann. Cardiol. Angeiol.*, 21: 379-388, 1972.

817. Bender, F., Modern drug therapy of arrhythmia, *Schweiz. Med. Wschr.*, 103: 272-276, 1973.

818. Bennett, W. M., Singer, I., and Coggins, C. H., Guide to drug usage in adult patients with impaired renal function, *JAMA*, 223: 991-997, 1973.

819. Berger, H., Fever: an unusual manifestation of epilepsy, *Postgrad. Med.*, 40: 479-481, 1966. *52*

820. Bergouignan, M., Antiepileptic drugs in the treatment of trigeminal neuralgia, *Presse Med.*, 78: 1832-1834, 1970.

821. Berlin, A., Agurell, S., Borga, O., Lund, L. and Sjoqvist, F., Micromethod for the determination of diphenylhydantoin in plasma and cerebrospinal fluid, *Scand. J. Clin. Invest.*, 29: 281-287, 1972.

822. Bernoulli, C., Diphenylhydantoin, *Schweiz. Med. Wschr.*, 100: 836, 1970.

823. Bernstein, J. D. and Johnson, S. L., Effects of diphenylhydantoin upon estrogen metabolism by liver *88* microsomes of DDT-treated Japanese quail, *Bull. Environ. Contam. Toxicol.*, 10: 309-314, 1973.

REFERENCES
Page

824. BERRY, D. J. and GROVE, J., Emergency toxicological screening for drugs commonly taken in overdose, *J. Chromatogr.*, 80: 205-219, 1973.

825. BHATT, G., VIJAYAN, N. and DREYFUS, P. M., Myotonia, *Calif. Med.*, 114: 16-22, 1971. *42*

826. BIGGER, J. T., JR., STEINER, C., and BURRIS, J. O., The effects of diphenylhydantoin on atrioventricular conduction in man, *Clin. Res.*, 15: 196, 1967.

827. BIGGER, J. T., SCHMIDT, D. H., and KUTT, H., A method for estimation of plasma diphenylhydantoin concentration, *Amer. Heart J.*, 77: 572-573, 1969.

828. BIGGER, J. T., WEINBERG, D. I., KOVALIK, T. W., HARRIS, P. D., CRANEFIELD, P. C., and Hoffman, B. F., *33* Effects of diphenylhydantoin on excitability and automaticity in the canine heart, *Circ. Res.*, 26: 1-15, 1970.

829. BIRKET-SMITH, E. and KROGH, E., Motor nerve conduction velocity during diphenylhydantoin intoxication, *Acta Neurol. Scand.*, 47: 265-271, 1971.

830. BISSETT, J. K., deSOYZA, N. D. B., KANE, J. J., and DOHERTY, J. E., Case studies: effect of diphenylhydantoin on induced aberrant conduction, *J. Electrocardiol.*, 7: 65-69, 1974.

831. BISSETT, J. K., deSOYZA, N. D. B., KANE, J. J., and MURPHY, M. L., Improved intraventricular conduction *26* of premature beats after diphenylhydantoin, *Amer. J. Cardiol.*, 33: 493-497, 1974.

832. BISSETT, J. K., KANE, J. J., deSOYZA, N., and DOHERTY, J., Effect of diphenylhydantoin on bundle branch block in man, *Clin. Res.*, 21: 405, 1973.

833. BISSETT, J. K., KANE, J., deSOYZA, N., and DOHERTY, J., Improved intraventricular conduction after diphenylhydantoin, *Circulation*, 48: 146, 1973.

834. BITTAR, E. E., CHEN, S. S., DANIELSON, B. G., and TONG, E. Y., An investigation of the action of diphenylhydantoin on sodium efflux in barnacle muscle fibres, *Acta Physiol. Scand.*, 89: 30-38, 1973.

835. BJERK, E. M. and HORNISHER, J. J., Narcolepsy: a case report and a rebuttal, *Electroenceph. Clin.* *52* *Neurophysiol.*, 10: 550-552, 1958.

836. BLACK, J. T., GARCIA-MULLIN, R., GOOD, E., and BROWN, S., Muscle rigidity in a newborn due to continuous peripheral nerve hyperactivity, *Arch. Neurol.*, 27: 413-425, 1972.

837. BLACK, N. D., The value of diphenylhydantoinate (Dilantin) in psychoses with convulsive disorders, *Psychiatr. Quart.*, 13: 711-720, 1939.

838. BLUM, M. R., McGILVERAY, I., BECKER, C. E., and RIEGELMAN, S., Clinical implications derived from pharmacokinetics of diphenylhydantoin (DPH), *Clin. Res.*, 19: 121, 1971.

839. BLUM, M., RIEGELMAN, S., and BECKER, C. E., Altered protein binding of diphenylhydantoin in uremic plasma, *New Eng. J. Med.*, 286: 109, 1972.

840. BLUMENKRANTZ, N. and ASBOE-HANSEN, G., Effect of diphenylhydantoin on connective tissue, *Acta Neurol. Scand.*, 50: 302-306, 1974.

841. BOCHNER, F., HOOPER, W. D., SUTHERLAND, J. M., EADIE, M. J. and TYRER, J. H., The renal handling of diphenylhydantoin and 5-(P-Hydroxyphenyl)-5-phenylhydantoin, *Clin. Pharmacol. Ther.*, 14: 791-796, 1973.

842. BOCHNER, F., HOOPER, W. D., TYRER, J. H., and EADIE, M. J., Effect of a delayed-action phenytoin preparation on blood phenytoin concentration, *J. Neurol. Neurosurg. Psychiat.*, 35: 682-684, 1972.

843. BOCHNER, F., HOOPER, W. D., SUTHERLAND, J. M., EADIE, M. J. and TYRER, J. H., Diphenylhydantoin concentrations in saliva, *Arch. Neurol.*, 31: 57-59, 1974.

844. BOCHNER, F., HOOPER, W. D., TYRER, J. H., and EADIE, M. J., Factors involved in an outbreak of phenytoin intoxication, *Epilepsy Abstracts*, 5: 245-246, 1971.

845. BOCHNER, F., HOOPER, W., TYRER, J., and EADIE, M., Clinical implications of certain aspects of diphenylhydantoin metabolism, *Proc. Aust. Assoc. Neurol.*, 9: 171-178, 1973.

846. BOGOCH, S. and DREYFUS, J., The broad range of use of diphenylhydantoin, bibliography and review, *The Dreyfus Medical Foundation*, 1970.

847. BOOKER, H. E., Serum concentrations of free diphenylhydantoin and their relationship to clinical intoxication, *Epilepsia*, 14: 96-97, 1973.

848. BOOKER, H. E., TORMEY, A., and Toussaint, J., Concurrent administration of phenobarbital and diphenylhydantoin: lack of an interference effect, *Neurology*, 21: 383-385, 1971.

849. BORGA, O., et al, Plasma protein binding of tricyclic antidepressants in man, *Psychopharm. Abs.*, 9: 500, 1970.

850. BORGA, O., GARLE, M., and GUTOVA, M., Identification of 5-(3, 4-dihydroxyphenyl)-5-phenylhydantoin as a metabolite of 5, 5-diphenylhydantoin (phenytoin) in rats and man, *Pharmacology*, 7: 129-137, 1972.

851. BORGSTEDT, A. D., BRYSON, M. F., YOUNG, L. W., and FORBES, G. B., Long-term administration of antiepileptic drugs and the development of rickets, *J. Pediat.*, 81: 9-15, 1972. (*cf.* Greenlaw, et al., *Clin. Res.*, 20: 56, 1972.)

852. BOROFSKY, L. G., LOUIS, S., and KUTT, H., Diphenylhydantoin in children, *Neurology*, 23: 967-972, 1973.

853. BORONDY, P., DILL, W. A., CHANG, T., BUCHANAN, R. A., and GLAZKO, A. J., Effect of protein binding on the distribution of 5, 5-diphenylhydantoin between plasma and red cells, *Ann. N. Y. Acad. Sci.*, 226: 82-87, 1973.

854. BOSE, B. C., GUPTA, S. S., and SHARMA, S., Effect of anticonvulsant drugs on the acetylcholine content in rat tissues, *Arch. Int. Pharmacodyn.*, 67: 254-261, 1958.

855. BOSHES, B. and ARIEFF, A. J., Clinical experience in the neurologic substance of pain, *Med. Clin. N. Amer.*, 52: 111-121, 1968.

856. BOSTON COLLABORATIVE DRUG SURVEILLANCE PROGRAM, Diphenylhydantoin side effects and serum albumin levels, *Clin. Pharmacol. Ther.*, 14: 529-532, 1973.

857. BOUDIN, G., PEPIN, B., DECROIX, G., and VERNANT, J. C., Diphenylhydantoin intoxication triggered by antituberculous treatment (2 cases), *Ann. Med. Intern.*, 122: 855-860, 1971.

858. BOUZARTH, W. F., The ABC's of emergency care of serious head injuries in industry, *Industr. Med. Surg.*, 39: 25-29, 1970.

859. BOWE, J. C., CORNISH, E. J., and DAWSON, M., Evaluation of folic acid supplements in children taking phenytoin, *Develop. Med. Child Neurol.*, 13: 343-354, 1971.

860. BOYD, D. L. and WILLIAMS, J. F., The effect of diphenylhydantoin (Dilantin) on the positive inotropic action of ouabain, *Amer. J. Cardiol.*, 23: 712-718, 1969.   *86*

861. BOYKIN, M. E. and HOOSHMAND, H., CSF and serum folic acid and protein changes with diphenylhydantoin treatment: laboratory and clinical correlations, *Neurology*, 20: 403, 1970.

862. BOYKIN, M. E., *In vivo* and *in vitro* association of 5, 5-diphenylhydantoin with brain subfractions, *Neurology*, 4: 392-393, 1974.   *93*

863. BOZZA, G. A., Normalization of intellectual development in the slightly brain-damaged, retarded child, *Paper presented at the 4th Italian National Congress on Child Neuropsychiatry*, Genoa, 1971.   *13*

864. BRAY, P. F., ELY, R. S., and KELLEY, V. C., Studies of 17-hydroxycorticosteroids VIII. Adrenocortical function in patients with convulsive disorders, *A.M.A. Arch. Neurol. Psychiat.*, 72: 583-590, 1954.

865. BRAY, P. F., ELY, R. S., ZAPATA, G., and KELLEY, V. C., Adrenocortical function in epilepsy I. The role of cortisol (hydrocortisone) in the mechanism and management of seizures, *Neurology*, 10: 842-846, 1960.

866. BRAY, P. F., KELLEY, V. C., ZAPATA, G., and ELY, R. S., Adrenocortical function in epilepsy II. The role of corticosterone in the mechanism and management of epilepsy, *Neurology*, 11: 246-250, 1961.

867. BRENA, S. and BONICA, J. J., Nerve blocks for managing pain in the elderly, *Postgrad. Med.*, 47: 215-220, 1970.

868. BRENNAN, R. W., DEHEJIA, H., KUTT, H., VEREBELY, K., and McDOWELL, F., Diphenylhydantoin intoxication attendant to slow inactivation of isoniazid, *Neurology*, 20: 687-693, 1970.

869. BRIEN, J. F. and INABA, T., Determination of low levels of 5,5 diphenylhydantoin in serum by gas liquid chromatography, *Epilepsy Abstracts*, 7: 198, 1974.

870. BRIGHT, N. H., Effect of diphenylhydantoin on proline and hydroxyproline excretion in the rat, *Proc. Soc. Exp. Biol. Med.*, 120: 463-465, 1965.

871. BRODDLE, W. D. and NELSON, S. R., The effect of diphenylhydantoin on brain P-creatine, *Fed. Proc.*, 28: 1771, 1969.

872. Brodows, R. G. and Campbell, R. G., Control of refractory fasting hypoglycemia in a patient with   *83*
suspected insulinoma with diphenylhydantoin, *J. Clin. Endocr.*, 38: 159-161, 1974.

873. Brown, G. L. and Wilson, W. P., Salicylate intoxication and the CNS with special reference to EEG findings, *Dis. Nerv. Syst.*, 32: 135-140, 1971.

874. Brown, J. M., Drug-associated lymphadenopathies with special reference to the Reed-Sternberg cell, *Med. J. Aust.*, 375-378, 1971.

875. Buchanan, R. A. and Allen, R. J., Diphenylhydantoin (Dilantin) and phenobarbital blood levels in epileptic children, *Neurology*, 21: 866-871, 1971.

876. Buchanan, R. A., Kinkel, A. W., Goulet, J. R., and Smith, T. C., The metabolism of diphenylhydantoin (Dilantin) following once-daily administration, *Neurology*, 22: 126-130, 1972.

877. Buchanan, R. A., Turner, J. L., Moyer, C. E., and Heffelfinger, J. C., Single daily dose of diphenylhydantoin in children, *J. Pediat.*, 83: 479-483, 1973.

878. Buchthal, F. and Lennox-Buchthal, M. A., Diphenylhydantoin, relation of anticonvulsant effect to concentration in serum, *Antiepileptic Drugs*, 193-209, Woodbury, D. M., Penry, J. K., and Schmidt, R. P., Eds., Raven Press, New York, 1972.

879. Buchthal, F. and Svensmark, O., Serum concentrations of diphenylhydantoin (phenytoin) and phenobarbital and their relation to therapeutic and toxic effects, *Psychiat. Neurol. Neurochir.*, 74: 117-136, 1971.

880. Burckhardt, D. and Sefidpar, M., Digitalis intoxication: contribution to diagnosis and therapy,   *86*
Schweiz. Rundschau. Med. (Praxis), 60: 1705-1711, 1971.

881. Buscaino, G. A., Labianca, O., Caruso, G., De Giacomo, P., and Ferrannini, E., Electromyographic   *42*
and muscular histoenzymatic findings in a patient with continuous muscular activity syndrome ("Neuromyotonia"), *Acta Neurol. (Naples)*, 25: 206-224, 1970.

882. Calne, D. B., The drug treatment of epilepsy, *Epilepsy Abstracts*, 6: 177, 1973.

883. Cantor, F. K., Phenytoin treatment of thalamic pain, *Brit. Med. J.*, 4: 590-591, 1972.   *36*

884. Caracta, A. R., Damato, A. N., Josephson, M. E., Ricciutti, M. A., Gallagher, J. J., and Lau, S. H., Electrophysiologic properties of diphenylhydantoin, *Circulation*, 47: 1234-1241, 1973.

885. Carnay, L. and Grundfest, S., Excitable membrane stabilization by diphenylhydantoin and calcium,   *62*
Neuropharmacology, 13: 1097-1108, 1974.

886. Caspary, W. F., Inhibition of intestinal calcium transport by diphenylhydantoin in rat duodenum, *Epilepsy Abstracts*, 6: 18, 1973.

887. Castleden, C. M. and Richens, A., Chronic phenytoin therapy and carbohydrate tolerance, *Lancet*, 966-967, 1973.

888. Chang, T. and Glazko, A. J., Diphenylhydantoin, biotransformation, *Antiepileptic Drugs*, 149-162, Woodbury, D. M., Penry, J. K., and Schmidt, R. P., Eds., Raven Press, New York, 1972.

889. Chang, T., Okerholm, R. A., and Glazko, A. J., A 3-0-methylated catechol metabolite of diphenylhydantoin (Dilantin) in rat urine, *Res. Communications Chem. Path. Pharmacol.*, 4: 13-23, 1972.

890. Chang, T., Savory, A. and Glazko, A. J., A new metabolite of 5, 5-diphenylhydantoin (Dilantin), *Biochem. Biophys. Res. Commun.*, 38: 444-449, 1970.

891. Cheng, P. T. H. and Staple, P. H., Effect of a dorsal dermal surgical wound on the chemical response of   *90*
rat abdominal skin to chronic administration of sodium diphenylhydantoin, *J. Dent. Res.*, 51: 131-143, 1972.

892. Cheng, T. O. and Damato, A. N., Dilantin in treatment and prevention of cardiac arrhythmias, *Amer. Heart J.*, 78: 285, 1969.

893. Chetchel, A. P., The influence of diphenine on the gum mucosa, *Epilepsy Abstracts*, 3: 203, 1970.

894. Chikhani, P., The use of 'diphenylhydantoin sodium' in the treatment of periodontal disease, *Actualities*   *51*
Odontostomat., 98: 1-8, 1972.

895. Choi, Y. K. and Kee, C. S., Induction of steroid 6 beta-hydroxylase by administration of diphenylhydantoin, *Chem. Abstracts*, 74: 123576C, 1971.

896. CHOI, Y., THRASHER, K., WERK, E. E., SHOLITON, L. J., and OLINGER, C., Effect of diphenylhydantoin on cortisol kinetics in humans, *J. Pharmacol. Exp. Ther.,* 176: 27-34, 1971. *80*

897. CHOKROVERTY, S. and RUBINO, F. A., Motor nerve conduction study in patients on long term diphenylhydantoin therapy: correlation with clinical states and serum levels of diphenylhydantoin, folate and cyanocobalamine, *Epilepsy Abstracts,* 7: 111, 1974.

898. CHOOVIVATHANAVANICH, P., WALLACE, E. M., and SCAGLIONE, P. R., Pseudolymphoma induced by diphenylhydantoin, *J. Pediat.,* 76: 621-623, 1970.

899. CHOU, C. C., KUIPER, D. H., and HSIEH, C. P., Effects of diphenylhydantoin on motility and compliance of the canine ileum and colon, *Gastroenterology,* 62: 734, 1972. *71*

900. CHRISKIE, H. W., du MESNIL DE ROCHEMONT, W., ETZRODT, H., GROSSER, K. D., Schulten, K. H., and STEINBRUCK, G., Influence of diphenylhydantoin and lidocaine on hemodynamics in patients with fixed-rate pacemakers, *Verh. Deutsch Ges. Inn. Med.,* 77: 960-963, 1971.

901. CHRISTIANSEN, C., RODBRO, P., and LUND, M., Effect of vitamin D on bone mineral mass in normal subjects and in epileptic patients on anticonvulsants: a controlled therapeutic trial, *Brit. Med. J.,* 208-209, 1973. (*cf.* CHRISTIANSEN, et al., *Brit. Med. J.,* 3: 738, 1972 and *Brit. Med. J.,* 4: 695, 1973.)

902. CHRISTIANSEN, J. and DAM, M., Influence of phenobarbital and diphenylhydantoin on plasma carbamazepine levels in patients with epilepsy, *Epilepsy Abstracts,* 7: 137, 1974.

903. CHRISTY, N. P. and HOFMANN, A. D., Effects of diphenylhydantoin upon adrenal cortical function in man, *Neurology,* 9: 245-248, 1959.

904. CHROBOK, F., Quantitative determination of phenytoin in biological material in the presence of phenobarbital and glutethimide, *Epilepsy Abstracts,* 5: 172, 1972.

905. CHUNG, E. K., The current status of digitalis therapy, *Modern Treatment,* 8: 643-714, 1971. *23*

906. CLARK, R. L., Kuhn, J. P., and Du JOVNE, C. A., Absence of rickets after chronic dilantin administration: experimental radiological observations in rats, *Invest. Radiol.,* 6: 152-154, 1971.

907. COBURN, R. F., Enhancement by phenobarbital and diphenylhydantoin of carbon monoxide production in normal man, *New Eng. J. Med.,* 283: 512-515, 1970.

908. COHEN, H., LANGENDORF, R., and PICK, A., Intermittent parasystole—mechanism of protection, *Circulation,* 48: 761-774, 1973.

909. COHEN, M. S., BOWER, R. H., FIDLER, S. M., JOHNSONBAUGH, R. E., and SODE, J., Inhibition of insulin release by diphenylhydantoin and diazoxide in a patient with benign insulinoma, *Lancet,* 40-41, 1973. *83*

910. COLE, P., Efficacy of oral diphenylhydantoin in reduction of premature ventricular contractions, *Clin. Pharmacol. Ther.,* 13: 137, 1972.

911. COLLAN, R., BOYD, W., and HATHAWAY, B., Effect of halothane on the liver of rats pretreated with diphenylhydantoin and norethindrone, *Scand. J. Clin. Lab. Invest.,* 25: 74, 1970.

912. CONN, H. L., JR., Mechanisms of quinidine action. *Mechanisms and Therapy of Cardiac Arrhythmias,* 594-596, Dreifus, L. S. and Likoff, W., Eds., Grune and Stratton, New York, 1966.

913. CONNERS, C. K., KRAMER, R., ROTHSCHILD, G. H., SCHWARTZ, L., and STONE, A., Treatment of young delinquent boys with diphenylhydantoin sodium and methyphenidate, *Arch. Gen. Psychiat.,* 24: 156-160, 1971.

914. CONNEY, A. H. and BURNS, J. J., Metabolic interactions among environmental chemicals and drugs, *Science,* 178: 576-586, 1972. *85*

915. CONNEY, A. H., JACOBSON, M., SCHNEIDMAN, K., and KUNTZMAN, R., Induction of liver microsomal cortisol 6 β-hydroxylase by diphenylhydantoin or phenobarbital: an explanation for the increased excretion of 6-hydroxycortisol in humans treated with these drugs, *Life Sci.,* 4: 1091-1098, 1965.

916. CONARD, G. J., HAAVIK, C. O., and FINGER, K. F., Binding of 5,5-diphenylhydantoin and its major metabolite to human and rat plasma proteins, *J. Pharm. Sci.,* 60: 1642-1646, 1971.

917. COOPER, R. G., GREAVES, M. S., and OWEN, G., Gas liquid chromatographic isolation, identification, and quantitation of some barbiturates, glutethimide, and diphenylhydantoin in whole blood, *Epilepsy Abstracts,* 6: 184, 1973.

REFERENCES

918. COSTA, P. J., GLASER, G. H., and BONNYCASTLE, D. D., Effects of diphenylhydantoin (Dilantin) on adrenal cortical function, *A.M.A. Arch. Neurol. Psychiat.*, 74: 88-91, 1955.

919. COVI, L. and UHLENHUTH, E. H., Methodological problems in the psychopharmacological study of the dangerous anti-social personality, *Proc. Int. Symposium on Aggressive Behavior Biochem. Pharmacol. Psychol. Sociol.*, 326-335, May, 1969.

920. COVINO, B. G., WRIGHT, R., and CHARLESON, D. A., Effectiveness of several antifibrillary drugs in the hypothermic dog, *Amer. J. Physiol.*, 121: 54-58, 1955.

921. CRANMER, M. F., Effect of diphenylhydantoin on storage of DDT in the rat, *Toxic Appl. Pharmacol.*, 17: 315, 1970. *85*

922. CRITCHLEY, E. M. R., CLARK, D. B., and WIKLER, A., An adult form of acanthocytosis, *Trans. Amer. Neurol. Assoc.*, 92: 132-137, 1967. *47*

923. CUAN-PEREZ, M. C. and ORTIZ, A., Comparative study of quinidine, propranolol and diphenylhydantoin for preventing recurrence in post-cardioversion auricular fibrillation, *Arch. Inst. Cardiol. Mex.*, 41: 278-284, 1971. *29*

924. CUDWORTH, A. G. and CUNNINGHAM, J. L., The effect of diphenylhydantoin on insulin response, *Clin. Sci. Molec. Med.*, 46: 131-136, 1974. *83*

925. CUMMINGS, N. P., ROSENBLOOM, A. L., KOHLER, W. C. and WILDER, B. J., Plasma glucose and insulin responses to oral glucose with chronic diphenylhydantoin therapy, *Pediatrics*, 51: 1091-1093, 1973.

926. CUNNINGHAM, J. L. and PRICE EVANS, D. A., Urinary D-glucaric acid excretion and acetanilide pharmacokinetics before and during diphenylhydantoin administration, *Europ. J. Clin. Pharmacol.*, 7: 387-391, 1974.

927. CURTIS, G. P., Experimental atrial fibrillation, *Univ. of Mich, Ann Arbor, Doctoral Thesis*, 1971. *32*

928. DACK, S., Antiarrhythmic agents in the treatment of ventricular tachycardia, *Mechanisms and Therapy of Cardiac Arrhythmias*, 312-320, Dreifus, L. S. and Likoff, W., Eds., Grune and Stratton, New York, 1966.

929. DALESSIO, D. J., Medical treatment of tic douloureux, *J. Chronic Dis.*, 19: 1043-1048, 1966.

930. DALTON, C. and VEREBELY, K., Hypotriglyceridemic activity of 5,5'-diphenyl-2-thiohydantoin (DPTH), *J. Pharmacol. Exp. Ther.*, 180: 484-491, 1971.

931. DALY, R. F. and SAJOR, E. E., Inherited tic douloureux, *Neurology*, 23: 937-939, 1973.

932. DAM, M. and CHRISTIANSEN, J., Evidence of drug action on serum level of carbamazepine, *Epilepsy Abstracts*, 7: 26, 1974.

933. DAM, M., Diphenylhydantoin, neurologic aspects of toxicity, *Antiepileptic Drugs*, 227-235, Woodbury, D. M., PENRY, J. K., and SCHMIDT, R. P. Eds., Raven Press, New York, 1972.

934. DAM, M., The density and ultrastructure of the Purkinje cells following diphenylhydantoin treatment in animals and man, *Acta Neurol. Scand.*, 48: 1-65, 1972.

935. DAMATO, A. N., BERKOWITZ, W. D., PATTON, R. D., and LAU, S. H., The effect of diphenylhydantoin on atrioventricular and intraventricular conduction in man, *Amer. Heart*, J.79: 51-56, 1970. *27*

936. DAMATO, A. N., Diphenylhydantoin: pharmacological and clinical use, *Progr. Cardiovasc. Dis.*, 12: 1-15, 1969.

937. DANCKWARDT-LILLIESTROM, G., GREVSTEN, S., and OLERUD, S., Investigation of effect of various agents on periosteal bone formation, *Upsala J. Med. Sci.*, 77: 125-128, 1972.

938. DANIEL, R., Psychiatric drug use and abuse in the aged, *Geriatrics*, 144-156, January, 1970. *14*

939. DANIELS, C., STEIN, A. A., and MOSS, G., The shock lung syndrome: anemia as a predisposing factor, *Surg. Forum*, 24: 1, 1973.

940. DANIELSON, B. G., BITTAR, E. E., CHEN, S. S. and TONG, E. Y., Diphenylhydantoin as a blocking agent of the proton-sensitive component of Na efflux in barnacle muscle fibers, *Life Sci.*, 10: 721-726, 1971.

941. DANZIG, R., Treatment of arrhythmias associated with acute myocardial infarction, *Nebraska Med. J.*, 56: 474-475, 1971. *86*

942. DAUBE, J. R. and PETERS, H. A., Hereditary essential myoclonus, *Arch. Neurol.*, 15: 587-594, 1966. *47*

943. Davies, J. E., Edmundson, W. F., Maceo, A., Irvin, G. L., Cassady, J., and Barquet, A., Reduction of pesticide residues in human adipose tissue with diphenylhydantoin, *Food Cosmet. Toxic.*, 9: 413-423, 1971. *85*

944. Davies, J. E., Pharmacological depletion of adipose pesticide residues, *Clin. Res.*, 19: 27, 1971. *85*

945. Davies, R. O., Diphenylhydantoin in angina pectoris, *Chest*, 66: 421-422, 1974.

946. Davis, J. N., Diphenylhydantoin for hiccups, *Lancet*, 1: 997, 1974. *46*

947. Dawson, K. P. and Jamieson, A., Value of blood phenytoin estimation in management of childhood epilepsy, *Arch. Dis. Child.*, 46: 386-388, 1971.

948. Dawson, K. P., Severe cutaneous reactions to phenytoin, *Arch. Dis. Child.*, 48: 239-240, 1973.

949. Day, H. W., Control and treatmetnt of arrhythmias, *Cardiovascular Therapy, The Art and The Science*, 289-291, Russek, H. I. and Zohman, B. L., Eds., The Williams & Wilkins, Co., Baltimore, 1971.

950. DeCastro, J. H. X., Acosta, M. L., Sica, R. E. P., and Guerico, N., Sensory and motor nerve conduction velocity in long-term diphenylhydantoin therapy, *Arq. Neuropsiquiat.*, 30: 215-220, 1972.

951. DeLuca, K., Masotti, R. E., and Partington, M. W., Altered calcium metabolism due to anticonvulsant drugs, *Develop. Med. Child Neurol.*, 14: 318-321, 1972.

952. Delaire, J., Moutet, H., and Talmant, J. C., Facial peripheric hemispasm and Paget's disease of bone, *Rev. Stomat. (Paris)*, 73: 601-612, 1972. *47*

953. Delgado, J. M. R. and Mihailovic, L., Use of intracerebral electrodes to evaluate drugs that act on the central nervous system, *Ann. N. Y. Acad. Sci.*, 64: 644-666, 1956. *12*

954. Delgado, J. M. R., Mora, F. and Sanguinetti, A. M., Reduction by diphenylhydantoin of after-discharges in the amygdala of stimulated rhesus monkey, *Personal Communication*, 1973. *12*

955. Den Hertog, A., The effect of diphenylhydantoin on the electronic component of the sodium pump in mammalian non-myelinated nerve fibers, *Europ. J. Pharmacol.*, 19: 94-97, 1972. *61*

956. Dent, E., Richens, A., Rowe, D. J. F., and Stamp, T. C. B., Osteomalacia with long-term anticonvulsant therapy in epilepsy, *Brit. Med. J.*, 4: 69-72, 1970.

957. Desjacques, P., Study of the diffusion of phenytoin through the cellophane membrane of the artificial kidney used on a patient suffering from uremia and epilepsy, *Epilepsy Abstracts*, 5: 220, 1972.

958. De Sousa, R. C. and Grosso, A., Effects of diphenylhydantoin on transport processes in frog skin (Rana ridibunda), *Epilepsy Abstracts*, 7: 111, 1974.

959. deWolff, F. A., Drug effects on intestinal epithelium, *Doctoral Thesis*, 1973.

960. Dhar, G. J., Peirach, C. A., Ahamed, P. N. and Howard, R. B., Diphenylhydantoin induced hepatic necrosis, *Postgrad. Med.*, 56: 128-129, 1974.

961. Diamond, B. and Yaryura-Tobias, J. A., The use of diphenylhydantoin in non-epileptic psychotics, *V World Congress of Psychiatry*, 1971. *15*

962. Diamond, W. D. and Buchanan, R. A., A clinical study of the effect of phenobarbital on diphenylhydantoin plasma levels, *J. Clin. Pharmacol.*, 306-311, 1970.

963. Diederich, K. W., Herzog, S. and Tielsen, I., Diphenylhydantoin: A comparative study on normal cats and animals intoxicated with digitalis glycosides, *Basic Research in Cardiology*, 69: 289-308, 1974. *86*

964. Dill, R. E., Adrenal cortical response in rats treated with diphenylhydantoin sodium, *Anat. Rec.*, 148: 366, 1964. *80*

965. Dill, W. A., Baukema, J., Chang, T., and Glazko, A. J., Colorimetric assay of 5,5-diphenylhydantoin (Dilantin) and 5 (p hydroxyphenyl) 5 phenylhydantoin, *Epilepsy Abstracts*, 4: 262, 1971.

966. Dill, W. A., Chucot, L., Chang, T., and Glazko, A. J., Simplified benzophenone procedure for determination of diphenylhydantoin in plasma, *Clin. Chem.*, 17: 1200-1201, 1971.

967. Dilman, V. M., Elivbaeva, G. V., Vishnevskii, A. S., Tsyrilina, E. V., and Bulovskaia, L. N., Justification of the use of diphenine (diphenylhydantoin) in oncologic practice, *Vop. Onkol.*, 17: 70-72, 1971.

968. Doe, W. F., Hoffbrand, A. V., Reed, P. I., and Scott, J. M., Jejunal pH and folic acid, *Brit. Med. J.*, 699-700, 1971.

REFERENCES

Page

969. DOHERTY, J. E., Digitalis glycosides. Pharmacokinetics and their clinical implications, *Ann. Intern. Med.*, 79: 229-238, 1973.   *86*

970. DOMINO, E. F. and OLDS, M. E., Effects of d-amphetamine, scopolamine, chlordiazepoxide and diphenyl-hydantoin on self-stimulation behavior and brain acetylcholine, *Psychopharmacologia (Berlin)*, 23: 1-16, 1972.

971. DOMZAL, T., Effect of diphenylhydantoin on clinical manifestations and excretion of 5-hydro-xyindoleacetic acid in Parkinson's disease, *Neurol. Neuochir. Pol.*, 6: 357-360, 1972.   *45*

972. DREIFUS, L. S. and WATANABE, Y., Current status of diphenylhydantoin, *Amer. Heart, J.*, 80: 709-713, 1970.

973. DREIFUS, L. S., de AZEVEDO, I. M. and WATANABE, Y., Electrolyte and antiarrhythmic drug interaction, *Amer. Heart J.*, 88: 95-107, 1974.

974. DREIFUS, L. S., Management of intractable atrial arrhythmias, *Mechanisms and Therapy of Cardiac Arrhythmias*, 205-210, Dreifus, L. S. and Likoff, W., Eds., Grune and Stratton, New York, 1966.

975. DREIFUS, L. S., Use of quinidine, procainamide and diphenylhydantoin, *Cariovascular Therapy, The Art and The Science*, 109-112, Russek, H. I. and Zohman, B. L., Eds., The Williams & Wilkins Co., Baltimore, 1971.

976. DREIFUSS, F. E. and SATO, S., Anticonvulsant drugs in clinical practice, *Drug Therapy*, 2: 9-22, 1972.

977. DREIFUSS, F. E., Diphenylhydantoin and visceral atony, *Drug Ther.*, 3: 101-102, 1973.

978. DRESSLER, W. E., ROSSI, G. V., and ORZECHOWSKI, R. F., Effect of several anticonvulsant drugs and procainamide against ouabain-induced cardiac arrhythmias in rabbits, *J. Pharm. Sci.*, 61: 133-134, 1972.   *86*

979. DRIESSEN, O. and EMONDS, A., Simultaneous determination of antiepileptic drugs in small samples of blood plasma by gas chromatography. Column technology and extraction procedure. *Epilepsy Abstracts*, 7: 203-204, 1974.

980. DRONAMRAJU, K. R., Epilepsy and cleft lip and palate, *Lancet*, 876-877, 1970.

981. DRY, J. and PRADALIER, A., Phenytoin intoxication during treatment combined with disulfiram, *Therapie*, 28: 799-802, 1973.

982. DUCKER, T. B., BLAYLOCK, R. L. D., and PEROT, P. L., JR., Emergency care of patients with cerebral injuries, *Postgrad. Med.*, 55: 102-110, 1974.

983. DUDLEY, W. H. C., JR., and WILLIAMS, J. G., Electroconvulsive therapy in delirium tremens, *Dig. Neurol. Psychiat.*, Series XL: 333, 1972.

984. DUJOVNE, C. A., CLARK, R., and LASAGNA, L., Calcium and CNS symptoms, *New Eng. J. Med.*, 281: 271-272, July, 1969.

985. EADIE, M. J., TYRER, J. H., and HOOPER, W. D., Aspects of diphenylhydantoin metabolism, *Proc. Aust. Assoc. Neurol.*, 7: 7-13, 1970.

986. EASTHAM, R. D. and JANCAR, J., Macrocytosis associated with anticonvulsant therapy, *Epilepsia*, 11: 275-280, 1970.

987. EDDY, J. D. and SINGH, S. P., Treatment of cardiac arrhythmias with phenytoin, *Brit. Med. J.*, 4: 270-273, 1969.   *24*

988. EDITOR, A guide to selection of a systemic antibacterial agent, *Drugs*, 4: 132-145, 1972.

989. EDITOR, Anticonvulsant drugs and hypocalcaemia, *Brit. Med. J.*, 4: 351, 1973.

990. EDITOR, Anticonvulsants or antiepileptics, *Behavioral Neuropsychiatry*, 3: 14-16, 1971.

991. EDITOR, Diphenylhydantoin for digitalis toxicity, *Postgrad. Med.*, 45: 244-245, 1969.   *86*

992. EDITOR, For tic douloureux, lasting relief, *Medical World News*, 14: 66-67, 1973.

993. EDITOR, Monitoring drug therapy, *Lancet*, 668, 1974.

994. EDITOR, Phenytoin and carbamazepine combined, *Brit. Med. J.*, 1: 113, 1974.

995. EDITOR, Some important interactions with anticonvulsant drugs, *J. International Res. Communication*, 2: 5-7, 1974.

996. EDITOR, Treatment of trigeminal neuralgia, *Brit. Med. J.*, 2: 583-584, 1972.

997. EDITORS, Panel discussion: hormones and fetal metabolism, *Clin. Pharmacol. Ther.*, 14: 742-747, 1973.

998. EDMUNDSON, W. F., DAVIES, J. E., MACEO, A., and MORGADE, C., Drug and environmental effects on DDT residues in human blood, *Southern Med. J.*, 63: 1440-1441, 1970. *85*

999. EDMUNDSON, W. F., FRAZIER, D. E., and MACEO, A., Sequential biochemical tests in persons taking pH phenytoin, *Indust..Med.*, 41: 7-11, 1972. *85*

1000. EHRNEBO, M., AGURELL, S., JALLING, B., and BOREUS, L. O., Age differences in drug binding by plasma proteins: studies on human fetuses, neonates and adults, *Europ. J. Clin. Pharmacol.*, 3: 189-193, 1971.

1001. EIPE, J., Drugs affecting therapy with anticoagulants, *Med. Clin. N. Amer.*, 56: 255-262, 1972.

1002. EISEN, A. A., WOODS, J. F., and SHERWIN, A. L., Peripheral nerve function in long-term therapy with diphenylhydantoin, *Neurology*, 24: 411-417, 1974.

1003. ELING, T. E., HARBISON, R. D., BECKER, B. A., and FOUTS, J. R., Diphenylhydantoin effect on neonatal and adult rat hepatic drug metabolism, *J. Pharmacol. Exp. Ther.*, 171: 127-134, 1970.

1004. ELING, T. E., HARBISON, R. D., BECKER, B. A., and FOUTS, J. R., Kinetic changes in microsomal drug metabolism with age and diphenylhydantoin treatment, *Europ. J. Pharmacol.*, 11: 101-108, 1970.

1005. ELLENBERGER, C., BURDE, R. M., and KELTNER, J. L., Acute optic neuropathy, *Arch. Opthal.*, 91: 435-438, 1974.

1006. ELLIOTT, T. H. and NATARAJAN, P. N., Infrared studies of hydantoin and its derivatives, *J. Pharm. Pharmacol.*, 19: 209-216, 1966.

1007. ELLIS, J. G. and DIMOND, E. G., Newer concepts of digitalis, *Amer. J. Cardiol.*, 17: 759-767, 1966. *86*

1008. ELSHOVE, J. and VAN ECK, J. H. M., Congenital malformations, cleft lip and palate in particular, in children of epileptic women, *Ned. Tijdschr. Geneesk.*, 115: 1371-1375, 1971. (*cf.* ELSHOVE, *Lancet*, 1074, 1969.)

1009. ELWOOD, J. C., RICHERT, D. A., and WESTERFELD, W. W., A comparison of hypolipidemic drugs in the prevention of an orotic acid fatty liver, *Biochem. Pharmacol.*, 21: 1127-1134, 1972.

1010. ERDEY, L., KAPLAR, L., TAKACS, J., and DESSOUKY, Y. M., Determination of hydantoins in pharmaceutical preparations by gas chromatography, *J. Chromatogr.*, 45: 63-67, 1969.

1011. ERICKSON, J. D. and OAKLEY, G. P., Seizure disorder in mothers of children with orofacial clefts: a case control study, *J. Pediat.*, 84: 244-246, 1974.

1012. ESCUETA, A. V. and APPEL, S. H., Brain synapses—an *in vitro* model for the study of seizures, *Arch. Intern. Med.*, 129: 333-344, 1972. *63*

1013. ESCUETA, A. V. and APPEL, S. H., The effects of electroshock seizures on potassium transport within synaptosomes from rat brain, *Epilepsy Abstracts*, 5: 205, 1972.

1014. ESCUETA, A. V. and APPEL, S. H., Diphenylhydantoin and potassium transport in isolated nerve terminals, *J. Clin. Invest.*, 50: 1977-1984, 1971.

1015. ESPOSITO-AVELLA, M. and MENNEAR, J. H., Studies on the protective effect of diphenylhydantoin against alloxan diabetes in mice, *Proc. Soc. Exp. Biol. Med.*, 142: 82-85, 1973. *84*

1016. EVANS, D. E. and GILLIS, R. A., Effect of diphenylhydantoin (DPH) on centrally induced vagal arrhythmias, *Pharmacologist*, 13: Abstract 188, 1971.

1017. EVENSON, M. A., JONES, P., and DARCEY, B., Simultaneous measurement of diphenylhydantoin and primidone in serum by gas-liquid chromatography, *Clin. Chem.*, 16: 107-110, 1970.

1018. FARISS, B. L. and LUTCHER, C. L., Diphenylhydantoin-induced hyperglycemia and impaired insulin release—effect of dosage, *Diabetes*, 20: 177-181, 1971.

1019. FDA, Anticonvulsant linked with birth defect risk, *FDA Drug Bulletin*, July, 1974.

1020. FEDRICK, J., Epilepsy and pregnancy: a report from the Oxford record linkage study, *Brit. Med. J.*, 2: 442-448, 1973.

1021. FERRARI, M. and FURLANUT, M., Effects of diphenylhydantoin on smooth muscle, *Arch. Int. Pharmacodyn.*, 203: 101-106, 1973. *72*

1022. FERRY, D. G., OWEN, D., and McQUEEN, E. G., The effect of phenytoin on the binding of pesticides to serum proteins, *Proc. Univ. Otago Med. School*, 50: 8-9, 1972. *85*

Page

1023. FERTZIGER, A. P. and DUNHAM, P. B., Diphenylhydantoin stimulation of potassium influx in isolated lobster axons, *Epilepsy Abstracts*, 5: 61, 1972.

1024. FERTZIGER, A. P., Brain extracellular space: some considerations on the role it plays in brain function, *Cond. Reflex*, 8: 224-232, 1973.

1025. FERTZIGER, A. P., LIUZZI, S. E., and DUNHAM, P. B., Diphenylhydantoin (Dilantin): stimulation of   *63*
potassium influx in lobster axons, *Brain Res.*, 33: 592-596, 1971.

1026. FERTZIGER, A. P., LYNCH, J. J., and STEIN, E. A., Modification of the morphine withdrawal syndrome in   *88*
rats, *Brain Res.*, 78: 331-334, 1974.

1027. FERTZIGER, A. P., STEIN, E. A., and LYNCH, J. J., Suppression of morphine-induced mania in cats,   *88*
Psychopharmacologia, 36: 185-187, 1974.

1028. FESTOFF, B. W. and APPEL, S. H., The effect of diphenylhydantoin on synaptosome metabolism, *Neurology*, 19: 300, 1969.

1029. FICA, V., PANAITESCU, G., MATRESCU, F., and POPESCU, E. A., Indications and limitations of anti-arrhythmic drugs, *Med. Intern.*, 23: 523-536, 1971.

1030. FINCHAM, R. W., SCHOTTELIUS, D. D., and SAHS, A. L., The influence of diphenylhydantoin on primidone metabolism, *Arch. Neurol.*, 30: 259-262, 1974.

1031. FINKLE, B. S., FOLTZ, R. L., and TAYLOR, D. M., A comprehensive GC-MS reference data system for toxicological and biomedical purposes, *J. Chromatogr. Sci.*, 12: 304-328, 1974.

1032. FISH, B., The "one child, one drug" myth of stimulants in hyperkinesis, *Arch. Gen. Psychiat.*, 25: 193-203, 1971.

1033. FISHER, D. and DIMINO, J. M., An alternative therapeutic approach for the heroin addict: diphenylhydan-   *19*
toin, *Personal Communication*, 1972.

1034. FISHER, D. D. and UNGERLEIDER, J. T., Grand mal seizures following ingestion of LSD, *Calif. Med.*, 106: 210-211, 1967.

1035. FORMBY, B., The *in vivo* and *in vitro* effect of diphenylhydantoin and phenobarbitone on K^+-activated phosphohydrolase and (NA^+K^+)-activated ATPase in particulate membrane fractions from rat brain, *J. Pharm. Pharmacol.*, 22: 81-85, 1970.

1036. FOUTS, J. R. and KUTT, H., Diphenylhydantoin, some studies on the biotransformation and interactions with some other drugs and chemicals, *Antiepileptic Drugs*, 163-168, Woodbury, D. M., Penry, J. K., and Schmidt, R. P., Eds., Raven Press, New York, 1972.

1037. FREIWALD, M. J., Prevention of complications of Herpes Zoster ophthalmicus with special reference to steroid therapy, *Eye, Ear, Nose and Throat Monthly*, 46: 444-450, 1967.

1038. FRENKEL, E. P., McCALL, M. S. and SHEEHAN, R. G., Cerebrospinal fluid folate, and vitamin B^{12} in anticonvulsant-induced magaloblastosis, *J. Lab. Clin. Med.*, 81: 105-115, 1973.

1039. FRIEDLANDER, W. J., Epilepsy—1973, *The Clinical Neurology Information Center*, The University of Nebraska Medical Center, 1-45, 1974.

1040. FRIEDMAN, A. P., An overview of chronic recurring headache, *Wisconsin Med. J.*, 71: 110-116, 1972.

1041. FRIEDMAN, A. P., Treatment of vascular headache, *International Encyclopedia of Pharmacology and Therapeutics*, Section 33, Vol. I: 225-251. Carpi, A., Ed., Pergamon Press, New York, 1972.

1042. FROMM, G. H., Pharmacological consideration of anticonvulsants, *Epilepsy Abstracts*, 2: 194, 1969.

1043. FROST, J. B., Mesoridazine and chlorpromazine in the treatment of alcohol withdrawal syndrome, *Canad. Psychiat. Assoc. J.*, 18: 385-387, 1973.

1044. GABLER, W. L. and HUBBARD, G. L., The metabolism of 5,5-diphenylhydantoin (DPH) in nonpregnant and pregnant Rhesus monkeys, *Arch. Int. Pharmacodyn.*, 203: 72-91, 1973.

1045. GABREELS, F. J. M., The influence of phenytoin on the Purkinje cell of the rat, *Epilepsy Abstracts*, 4: 131-132, 1971.

1046. GALLAGHER, B. B., BAUMEL, I. P., MATTSON, R. H., and WOODBURY, S. G., Primidone, diphenylhydantoin and phenobarbital: aspects of acute and chronic toxicity, *Neurology*, 23: 145-149, 1973.

1047. GAMSTORP, I., MEEUWISSE, G., and TRYDING, N., Tryptophan loading test in convulsive disorders, *Acta Paediat. Scand.*, 55: 656-657, 1966.

1048. GARDNER-MEDWIN, D., Why should we measure serum levels of anticonvulsant drugs in epilepsy?, *Clinical Electroencephalograpy*, 4: 132-134, 1973.

1049. GARDNER, C. R. and WEBSTER, R. A., The effect of some anticonvulsant drugs on leptazol and bicuculline induced acetylcholine efflux from rat cerebral cortex, *Brit. J. Pharmacol.*, 47: 652P, 1973.

1050. GARRETTSON, L. K. and CURLEY, A., Dieldrin—studies in a poisoned child, *Arch. Environ. Health*, 19: 814-822, 1969.

1051. GARRETTSON, L. K., Pharmacology of anticonvulsants, *Pediat. Clin. N. Amer.*, 19: 179-191, 1972.

1052. GATTENLOHNER, W. and SCHNEIDER, K. W., The effect of diphenylhydantoin on hemodynamics,   *23* *Munchen Med. Wschr.*, 11: 2561-2566, 1969.

1053. GAUCHEL, F. D., LEHR, H. J., GAUCHEL, G., and VON HARNACK, G. A., Diphenylhydantoin in children, *Deutsch Med. Wschr.*, 98: 1391-1396, 1973.

1054. GAUCHEL, G., GAUCHEL, F. D., and BIRKOFER, L., A micromethod for the determination of phenytoin in blood by high speed liquid chromatography, *Epilepsy Abstracts*, 6: 210, 1973.

1055. GAVRILESCU, S., POP, T., and GOIA, E., On a case of supraventricular paroxysmal tachycardia resistant to treatment. Transitory conversion into atrial fibrillation by rapid atrial electric stimulation, *Med. Intern (Bucur)*, 24: 1393-1400, 1972.

1056. GEBAUER, D., Prevention and therapy of cardiac rhythm disorders. Experiences with a diphenylhydantoin-meprobamate preparation (cusitan), *Munchen Med. Wschr.*, 113: 436-440, 1971.

1057. GEGICK, C. G., DANOWSKI, T. S., KHURANA, R. C., VIDALON, C., NOLAN, S., STEPHAN, T., CHAE, S., and WINGARD, L., Hyperostosis frontalis interna and hyperphosphatasemia, *Ann. Intern. Med.*, 79: 71-75, 1973.

1058. GEHRES, L. D., RANDALL, C. L., RICCIO, D. C., and VARDARIS, R. M., Attenuation of hypothermic   *89* retrograde amnesia produced by pharmacologic blockage of brain seizures, *Physiol. Behav.*, 10: 1011-1017, 1973.

1059. GERBER, N., LYNN, R., and OATES, J., Acute intoxication with 5,5-diphenylhydantoin associated with impairment of biotransformation, *Ann. Intern. Med.*, 77: 765-771, 1972.

1060. GERBER, N., SEIBERT, R. A. and THOMPSON, R. M., Identification of a catechol glucuronide metabolite of 5,5 diphenylhydantoin (DPH) in rat bile by gas chromatography (GC) and mass spectrometry (MS), *Epilepsy Abstracts*, 7: 80, 1974.

1061. GERBER, N., WELLER, W. L., LYNN, R., RANGNO, R. E., SWEETMAN, B. J., and BUSH, M. T., Study of dose-dependent metabolism of 5,5-diphenylhydantoin in the rat using new methodology for isolation and quantitation of metabolites *in vivo* and *in vitro*, *J. Pharmacol. Exp. Ther.*, 178: 567-579, 1971.

1062. GERICH, J. E., CHARLES, M. A., LEVIN, S. R., FORSHAM, P. H., and GRODSKY, G. M., *In vitro* inhibition of   *84* pancreatic glucagon secretion by diphenylhydantoin, *J. Clin. Endocr.*, 35: 823-824, 1972.

1063. GERLINGS, E. D. and GILMORE, J. P., Some cardiac effects of diphenylhydantoin, *Acta Physiol. Pharmacol. Neerl.*, 15: 461-468, 1969.

1064. GERMAN, J., KOWAL, A., and EHLERS, K. H., Trimethadione and human teratogenesis, *Teratology*, 3: 349-362, 1970.

1065. GERSON, C. D., HEPNER, G. W., BROWN, N., COHEN, N., HERBERT, V., and JANOWITZ, H. D., Inhibition by diphenylhydantoin of folic absorption in man, *Gastroenterology*, 63: 246-251, 1972.

1066. GERZ, H. O., Dilantin against "painful touching" (dysthesia), *Physician's Drug Manual*, 3: 144, 1972.   *37*

1067. GETTES, L. S., The electrophysiologic effects of antiarrhythmic drugs, *Amer. J. Cardiol.*, 28: 526-535, 1971.

1068. GHARIB, H. and MUNOZ, J. M., Endocrine manifestations of diphenylhydantoin therapy, *Metabolism*, 23: 515-524, 1974.

1069. GIANELLY, R. E. and HARRISON, D. C., Drugs used in the treatment of cardiac arrhythmias, *Disease-A-Month*, 25-32, January, 1969.

1070. GIBSON, K. and HARRIS, P., Diphenylhydantoin and human myocardial microsomal (Na$^+$, K$^+$)-ATPase, *Biochem. Biophys. Res. Commun.*, 35: 75-78, 1969.

REFERENCES

Page

1071. GILBERT, J. C., GRAY, P., and HEATON, G. M., Anticonvulsant drugs and brain glucose, *Biochem. Pharmacol.*, 20: 240-243, 1971. *69*

1072. GILLIS, R. A. and RAINES, A., A comparison of the cardiovascular effects of diphenylthiohydantoin and diphenylhydantoin, *Europ. J. Pharmacol.*, 23: 13-18, 1973.

1073. GIMENEZ-ROLDAN, S. and ESTEBAN, A., Orbicularis oculi "myotonia" in hypothyroid myopathy, *Europ. Neurol.*, 9: 44-55, 1973. *43*

1074. GINWALLA, T. M. S., GOMES, B. C., and NAYAK, R. P., Management of gingival hyperplasia in patients receiving Dilantin therapy, *J. Indian Dent. Assn.*, 39: 124-126, 1967.

1075. GLASER, G. H., Diphenylhydantoin, toxicity, *Antiepileptic Drugs*, 219-226, WOODBURY, D. M., PENRY, J. K., and SCHMIDT, R. P. Eds., Raven Press, New York, 1972. (*cf.* ADELOYE, et al., *Ghana Med. J.*, 10: 56, 1971, BOSSO AND CHUDZIK, *Drug Intel. & Clin. Pharma.*, 7: 336, 1973, GREENBERG, et al., *Epilepsy Abstracts*, 4: 151, 1971 and WATTS, *Pediatrics*, 30: 592, 1962.) *54*

1076. GLAZKO, A. J. and CHANG, T., Diphenylhydantoin, absorption, distribution and excretion, *Antiepileptic Drugs*, 127-136, Woodbury, D. M., Penry, J. K., and Schmidt, R. P., Eds., Raven Press, New York, 1972.

1077. GLAZKO, A. J., Diphenylhydantoin, chemistry and methods for determination, *Antiepileptic Drugs*, 103-112, Woodbury, D. M., Penry, J. K., and Schmidt, R. P., Eds., Raven Press, New York, 1972.

1078. GLAZKO, A. J., Diphenylhydantoin, *Epilepsy Abstracts*, 6: 184, 1973.

1079. GODFRAIND, T., LESNE, M., and POUSTI, A., The action of diphenylhydantoin upon drug binding, ionic effects and inotropic action of ouabain, *Arch. Int. Pharmacodyn.*, 191: 66-73, 1971. *86*

1080. GOEBEL, R. W., Sodium diphenylhydantoin association with oral healing, *J. Oral Surg.*, 30: 191-195, 1972. *52*

1081. GOLDBERG, M. A., and TODOROFF, T., Binding of diphenylhydantoin to brain protein, *Epilepsy Abstracts*, 7: 112, 1974.

1082. GOLDBERG, M. A. and TODOROFF, T., Diphenylhydantoin binding to brain fractions, *Neurology*, 22: 410, 1972. *94*

1083. GOLDBERG, M. E. and CIOFALO, V. B., Effect of diphenylhydantoin sodium and chlordiazepoxide alone and in combination on punishment behavior, *Psychopharmacologia (Berlin)*, 14: 233-239, 1969.

1084. GOLDSTEIN, F. J., Continuing education via pharmatapes: Digitalis I. A basic pharmacological review, *Amer. J. Pharm.*, 145: 135-141, 1973. *86*

1085. GOLDSTEIN, R. E., PENZOTTI, S. C., KUEHL, K. S., PRINDLE, K. H., HALL, C. A., TITUS, E. O., and EPSTEIN, S. E., Correlation of antiarrhythmic effects of diphenylhydantoin with digoxin-induced changes in myocardial contractility, sodium-potassium adenosine triphosphatase activity, and potassium efflux, *Circ. Res.*, 33: 175-182, 1973. *33*

1086. GORDON, E., Respiratory control after acute head injury, *Lancet*, 483, 1973.

1087. GORDON, P., Aging: a search for drug-modifiable degeneracy in the polyribosomes of brain, *Proc. 8th Int. Cong. Geront.*, 1: 4pp., 1969.

1088. GORDON, P., CALLAGHAN, O., and DOTY, B., Diphenylhydantoin effects on nucleic acid biochemistry learning and neoplasm, *Pharmacologist*, 10: 169, 1968. *89*

1089. GORDON, P., Molecular approaches to the drug enhancement of deteriorated functioning in the aged, *Advances Geront. Res.*, 3: 199-248, 1971.

1090. GORDON, P., Rational chemotherapy for aging, *Postgrad. Med.*, 40: 152-155, 1970.

1091. GORDON, P., TOBIN, S. S., DOTY, B., and NASH, M., Drug effects on behavior in aged animals and man: diphenylhydantoin and procainamide, *J. Geront.*, 23: 434-444, 1968.

1092. GOSSEL, T. A. and Mennear, J. H., Inhibition of alloxan-induced diabetes by diphenylhydantoin sodium, *Pharmacologist*, 13: 238, 1971. *84*

1093. GOSSEL, T. A., On the mechanism of diphenylhydantoin protection against alloxan-induced diabetes mellitus in mice, *Dissertation Abstracts*, 33: 2729B, 1972.

1094. GOTTSCHALK, L. A., COVI, L., ULIANA, R., and BATES, D. E., Effects of diphenylhydantoin on anxiety and hostility in institutionalized prisoners, *Compr. Psychiat.*, 14: 503-511, 1973.

1095. GOUDIE, J. H. and BURNETT, D., A gas chromatographic method for the simultaneous determination of phenobarbitone, primidone and phenytoin in serum using a nitrogen detector, *Epilepsy Abstracts*, 6: 187, 1973.

1096. GRANT, R. H. E. and STORES, O. P. R., Folic acid in folate-deficient patients with epilepsy, *Brit. Med. J.*, 4: 644-648, 1970.

1097. GREEN, R. S. and RAU, J. H., Treatment of compulsive eating disturbances with anticonvulsant medication, *Amer. J. Psychiat.*, 131: 428-432, 1974.   *18*

1098. GREENBAUM, D. S., FERGUSON, R. K., KATER, L. A., KUIPER, D. H., and ROSEN, L. W., A controlled therapeutic study of the irritable-bowel syndrome, *New Eng. J. Med.*, 288: 13-16, 1973.   *47*

1099. GREENBERG, C. and PAPPER, E. M., The indications for gasserian ganglion block for trigeminal neuralgia, *Anesthesiology*, 31: 566-573, 1969.

1100. GREENBERG, I. M., Cerebral dysfunction in general psychiatric office practice, *Dis. Nerv. Syst.*, 33: 637-644, 1972.

1101. GREENGARD, O. and McILWAIN, H., Anticonvulsants and the metabolism of separated mammalian cerebral tissues, *Biochem. J.*, 61: 61-68, 1955.

1102. GROB, P. J. and HEROLD, G. E., Immunological abnormalities and hydantoins, *Brit. Med. J.*, 2: 561-563, 1972.

1103. GRUENER, R. P. and STERN, L. Z., Diphenylhydantoin reverses membrane effects in steroid myopathy, *Nature New Bio.*, 235: 54-55, 1972.   *71*

1104. GUDMUNDSON, C. and LIDGREN, L., Does diphenylhydantoin accelerate healing of fractures in mice, *Acta Orthop. Scand.*, 44: 640-649, 1973.   *90*

1105. GUZEK, J. W., RUSSELL, J. T., and THORN, N. A., Inhibition by diphenylhydantoin of vasopressin release from isolated rat neurohypophyses, *Acta Pharmacol. et Toxicol.*, 34: 1-4, 1974.   *81*

1106. HAAN, D., *Diagnosis and therapy of cardiac arrhythmia and acute heart disease*, Medizinisch Literarische Verlagsgesellschaft mbH, Uelzen, Germany, 1973.

1107. HADDAD, R. I., Positive EEG spike activity in sleep, *JAMA*, 229: 1282, 1974.

1108. HADFIELD, M. G. and BOYKIN, M. E., Effect of diphenylhydantoin administered *in vivo* on 3H-1-norepinephrine uptake in synaptosomes, *Res. Commun. Chem. Pathol. Pharmacol.*, 7: 209-212, 1974.   *78*

1109. HADFIELD, M. G., Uptake and binding of catecholamines—effect of diphenylhydantoin and a new mechanism of action, *Arch. Neurol.*, 26: 78-84, 1972.   *78*

1110. HAFT, J. I., RICCIUTTI, M. A. and DAMATO, A. N., Effects of IV diphenylhydantoin (DPH) on coronary blood flow and oxygen utilization of the heart, *Clinical Research*, 15: 204, 1967.

1111. HAGEN, H., Treatment of cardiac arrhythmias with diphenylhydantoin, *Deutsch Med. Wschr.*, 96: 380-384, 1971.

1112. HAGHSHENASS, M. and RAO, D. B., Serum folate levels during anticonvulsant therapy with diphenylhydantoin, *J. Amer. Geriat. Soc.*, 21: 275-277, 1973.

1113. HAHN, T. J., HENDIN, B. A., SCHARP, C. R., and HADDAD, J. G., JR., Effect of chronic anticonvulsant therapy on serum 25-hydroxycalciferol levels in adults, *New Eng. J. Med.*, 287: 900-909, 1972.

1114. HAIAT, R., CHAPELLE, M., BENAIM, R., WITCHITZ, S., and CHICHE, P., Disappearance of an intraventricular conduction disorder under diphenylhydantoin, *Sem. Hop. Paris*, 47: 2957-2964, 1971.   *86*

1115. HALL, W. B., Prevention of Dilantin hyperplasia: a preliminary report, *Bull. Acad. Gen. Dent.*, 20-25, 1969.

1116. HALLAQ, I. Y. and HARRIS, J. D., The syndrome of postherpetic neuralgia: complication and an approach to therapy, *J. Amer. Osteopath. Assoc.*, 68: 1265-1267, 1969.   *37*

1117. HALPERN, L. M. and JULIEN, R. M., Augmentation of cerebellar Purkinje cell discharge rate after diphenylhydantoin, *Epilepsy Abstracts*, 5: 236-237, 1972.

1118. HANCOCK, J. C. and BEVILACQUA, A. R., Temporal lobe dysrhythmia and impulsive or suicidal behavior, *Southern Med. J.*, 64: 1189-1193, 1971.

1119. HANDLEY, A. J., Phenytoin tolerance tests, *Brit. Med. J.*, 3: 203-204, 1970.

REFERENCES

Page

1120. HANSEN, H. W. and WAGENER, H. H., Sodium diphenylhydantoin for the treatment of cardiac arrhythmias, *Munchen Med. Wschr.*, 111: 417-421, 1969. — *27*

1121. HANSEN, H. W. and WAGENER, H. H., Diphenylhydantoin in the treatment of heart failure, *Deutsch. Med. Wschr.*, 96: 1866-1873, 1971. — *23*

1122. HANSEN, H. W. and WAGENER, H. H., Experimental studies on the influence of diphenylhydantoin glycoside effects on the heart, *Herz Kreislauf Zeitschrift Fur Kardiologie und Angiologie in Klinik und Praxis*, 6: 69-72, 1974. — *34*

1123. HANSEN, H. W., MARQUORT, B., and PELZ, W., Indications for phenytoin in cardiac arrhythmias, *Deutsch. Med. Wschr.*, 99: 638-642, 1974.

1124. HANSEN, J. M., SIERSBAEK-NIELSEN, K. and SKOVSTED, L., Effect of diphenylhydantoin on the metabolism of carbamazepine-induced acceleration of dicoumarol in man, *Acta Med. Scand.*, 189: 15-19, 1971.

1125. HANSEN, J. M., SKOVSTED, L., LAURIDSEN, U. BIRK, KIRKEGAARD, C., and SIERSBAEK-NIELSEN, K., The effect of diphenylhydantoin on thyroid function, *J. Clin. Endocrinol. Metab.*, 39: 785-786, 1974.

1126. HANSOTIA, P. and KERAN, E., Dilantin binding by red blood cells of normal subjects, *Neurology*, 24: 575-578, 1974.

1127. HANSTEN, P. D., Diphenylhydantoin drug interactions, *Hosp. Formulary Manage.*, 4: 28-29, 1969.

1128. HAQUE, N., THRASHER, K., WERK, E. E., JR., KNOWLES, H. C., JR., and SHOLITON, L. J., Studies on dexamethasone metabolism in man: effect of diphenylhydantoin, *J. Clin. Endocr.*, 34: 44-50, 1972. — *81*

1129. HARBISON, R. D. and BECKER, B. A., Effect of phenobarbital and SKF 525A pretreatment on diphenylhydantoin teratogenicity in mice, *J. Pharmacol. Exp. Ther.*, 175: 283-288, 1970.

1130. HARBISON, R. D., ELING, T. E., and BECKER, B. A., Effects of diphenylhydantoin on neonatal rat liver drug metabolizing enzymes, *Fed. Proc.*, 28(2): 1969.

1131. HARRIS, M., JENKINS, M. V. and WILLS, M. R., Phenytoin inhibition of parathyroid hormone induced bone resorption *in vitro*, *Brit. J. Pharmac.*, 50: 405-408, 1974. — *78*

1132. HARRISON, D. C., KERBER, R. E., and ALDERMAN, E. L., Pharmacodynamics and clinical use of cardiovascular drugs after cardiac surgery, *Amer. J. Cardiol.*, 26: 385-393, 1970.

1133. HART, B. L., Feline behavior, *Feline Practice*, 3: 8-10, 1973.

1134. HARTSHORN, E. A., Interactions of cardiac drugs, *Drug Intell. Clin. Pharm.*, 4: 272-275, 1970.

1135. HARTSHORN, E. A., Pyrazolone derivatives (antipyrine, aminopyrine, phenylbutazone, oxyphenbutazone), *Drug Intelligence Clincial Pharmacy*, 6: 6-10, 1972.

1136. HASBANI, M., PINCUS, J. H. and LEE, S. H., Diphenylhydantoin and calcium movement in lobster nerves, *Arch. Neurol.*, 31: 250-254, 1974.

1137. HATCH, R. C. and FISCHER, R., Cocaine elicited behavior and toxicity in dogs pretreated with synaptic blocking agents, morphine, or diphenylhydantoin, *Epilepsy Abstracts*, 6: 209, 1973.

1138. HATTWICK, M. A. W., WEIS, T. T., STECHSCHULTE, C. J., BAER, G. M., and GREGG, M. B., Recovery from rabies: a case report, *Ann. Intern. Med.*, 76: 931-942, 1972. — *53*

1139. HAWARD, L. R. C., Effects of sodium diphenylhydantoinate and pemoline upon concentration: a comparative study, *Drugs and Cerebral Function*, 103-120, Smith, W. L., Ed., Charles C. Thomas, 1970. — *16*

1140. HAWARD, L. R. C., Effects of DPH (sodium diphenylhydantoinate) upon concentration in pilots, *Rev. Med. Aeronautique Spatiale*, 12: 372-374, 1973. — *17*

1141. HAWARD, L. R. C., The effect of phenytoin-aided autogenic training on stress threshold, *Int. Congress for Psychosomatic Med. and Hypnosis*, Kyoto, Japan, July 12-14, 1967.

1142. HAWARD, L. R. C., Effects of sodium diphenylhydantoin upon concentration, *Bulletin Brit. Psychol. Soc.*, 22: 50, 1969.

1143. HEDGER, R. W., The conservative management of acute oliguric renal failure, *Med. Clin. N. Amer.*, 55: 121-135, 1971.

1144. HEINEMANN, U. and LUX, H. D., Effects of diphenylhydantoin on extracellular (K+) in cat cortex, *Electroenceph. Clin. Neurophysiol.*, 34: 735, 1973.

1145. HELFANT, R., SCHERLAG, B., and DAMATO, A., The interaction of procaine amide and diphenylhydantoin on cardiac conductivity and automaticity, *Clin. Res.*, 15: 206, 1967.

1146. HENDRICKS, G. L., JR., BARNES, W. T., and HOOD, H. L., Seven-year "cure" of lung cancer with metastasis to the brain, *JAMA*, 220: 127, 1972.

1147. HEPNER, G. W., ALEDORT, L. M., GERSON, C. D., COHEN, N., HERBERT, V., and JANOWITZ, H. D., Inhibition of intestinal ATPase by diphenylhydantoin and acetazolamide, *Clin. Res.*, 18: 382, 1970.

1148. HERBINGER, W., Result report of a control by an apparatus of 208 myocardial infarct patients in an intensive care station, *Wien. Med. Wschr.*, 121: 518-522, 1971.

1149. HERMANSEN, K., Antifibrillatory effect of some beta-adrenergic receptor blocking agents determined by a new test procedure in mice, *Acta Pharmacolgica*, 28: 17-27, 1969.

1150. HINKHOUSE, A., Craniocerebral trauma, *Amer. J. Nurs.*, 73: 1719-1722, 1973.

1151. HOBSON, J. D. and ZETTNER, A., Digoxin serum half-life following suicidal digoxin poisoning, *JAMA*, 223: 147-149, 1973.   *86*

1152. HODGSON, E. R. and REESE, H. H., Clinical experiences with dilantin in epilepsies, *Wis. Med. J.*, 38: 968-971, 1939.

1153. HOEFER, P. F. A., COHEN, S. M., and GREELEY, D. McL., Paroxysmal abdominal pain—a form of epilepsy in children, *JAMA*, 147: 1-6, 1951.

1154. HOFELDT, F. D., DIPPE, S. E., LEVIN, S. R., KARAM, J. H., BLUM, M. R., and FORSHAM, P. H., Effects of diphenylhydantoin upon glucose-induced insulin secretion in three patients with insulinoma, *Diabetes*, 23: 192-198, 1974.   *82*

1155. HOGG, P. S., Three cases of 'restless legs' or 'Ekbom's syndrome' as seen in general practice, *Practitioner*, 209: 82-83, 1972.   *44*

1156. HOLCOMB, R., LYNN, R., HARVEY, B., SWEETMAN, B. J., and GERBER, N., Intoxication with 5,5-diphenyl-hydantoin (Dilantin), *J. Pediat.*, 80: 627-632, 1972.

1157. HOLDAWAY, P. A., Effects of amino-glutethimide and diphenylhydantoin sodium on the rat adrenal cortex, *Proc. Indiana Acad. Sci.*, 77: 427-433, 1968.   *80*

1158. HOMMES, O. R. and OBBENS, E. A., The epileptogenic action of Na-folate in the rat, *J. Neurol. Sci.*, 16: 271-281, 1972.

1159. HONDA, Y., PODOS, S. M., and BECKER, B., The effect of diphenylhydantoin on the electroretinogram of rabbits. I. Effect of concentration, *Invest. Ophthal.*, 12: 567-572, 1973.

1160. HONDA, Y., PODOS, S. M., and BECKER, B., The effect of diphenylhydantoin on the electroretinogram of rabbits. II. Effects of hypoxia and potassium, *Invest. Ophthal.*, 12: 573-578, 1973.   *68*

1161. HOOPER, W. D., SUTHERLAND, J. M., BOCHNER, F. et al., The effect of certain drugs on the plasma protein binding of phenytoin, *Epilepsy Abstracts*, 7: 112, 1974.

1162. HOPF, H. C. and KAUER, H., Effect of phenytoin on the excitable cell membrane, *Epilepsy Abstracts*, 4: 89, 1971.

1163. HOUBEN, P. F. M., HOMMES, O. R., and KNAVEN, P. J. H., Anticonvulsant drugs and folic acid in young mentally retarded epileptic patients, *Epilepsia*, 12: 235-247, 1971.

1164. HOUCK, J. C., CHENG, R. F., and WATERS, M. D., Diphenylhydantoin, effects on connective tissue and wound repair, *Antiepileptic Drugs*, 267-273, Woodbury, D. M., Penry, J. K., and Schmidt, R. P., Eds., Raven Press, New York, 1972.   *90*

1165. HOUCK, J. C., CHENG, R. F., and WATERS, M. D., The effect of Dilantin upon fibroblast proliferation, *Proc. Soc. Exp. Biol. Med.*, 139: 969-981, 1972.

1166. HOUGHTON, G. W. and RICHENS, A., Inhibition of phenytoin metabolism by sulthiame in epileptic patients, *Brit. J. Clin. Pharmacol.*, 1: 59-66, 1974.

1167. HOUGHTON, G. W. and RICHENS, A., Rate of elimination of tracer doses of phenytoin at different steady state serum phenytoin concentrations in epileptic patients, *Brit. J. Clin. Pharmacol.* 1: 155-161, 1974.

1168. HOUGHTON, G. W., LATHAM, A. N., and RICHENS, A., Difference in the central actions of phenytoin and phenobarbitone in man, measured by critical flicker fusion threshold, *Europ. J. Clin. Pharmacol.*, 6: 57-60, 1973.   *88*

REFERENCES

1169. HUESSY, H. R., Study of the prevalence and therapy of the choreatiform syndrome or hyperkinesis in rural Vermont, *Acta Paedopsychiat.,* 34: 130-135, 1967.

1170. HUFFMAN, D. H. and AZARNOFF, D. L., The use of digitalis, *Ration. Drug Ther.,* 8: 1-7, 1974. *86*

1171. HUGHES, R. C. and MATTHEWS, W. B., Pseudo-myotonia and myokymia, *J. Neurol. Neurosurg. Psychiat.,* *41* 32: 11-14, 1969.

1172. HUISMAN, J. W., VAN HEYCOP TEN HAM, M. W., and VAN ZIJL, C. H. W., Influence of ethylphenacemide on serum levels of other anti-epileptic drugs, *Epilepsia,* 11: 207-215, 1970.

1173. HUMPHRIES, J. O., New methods for the prevention and treatment of ventricular arrhythmias, *Maryland Med. J.,* 17: 75-76, 1968.

1174. HUNNINGHAKE, D. B., Drug interactions, *Postgrad. Med.,* 47: 71-75, 1970.

1175. HUNTER, J., MAXWELL, J. D., STEWART, D. A., PARSONS, V., and WILLIAMS, R., Altered calcium metabolism in epileptic children on anticonvulsants, *Brit. Med. J.,* 202-204, 1971. (*cf.* HAHN, et al., *Clin. Res.,* 21: 626, 1973 and HERMAN AND PIPPENGER, *Neurology,* 23: 437, 1973.)

1176. IBER, F. L., Prevention of alcohol withdrawal seizures, *JAMA,* 221: 608, 1972.

1177. IDE, C. H. and WEBB, R. W., Penetrating transorbital injury with cerebrospinal orbitorrhea, *Amer. J. Ophthal.,* 71: 1037-1039, 1971.

1178. IDESTROM, C. M., SCHALLING, D., CARLQUIST, U., and SJOQVIST, F., Acute effects of diphenylhydantoin in relation to plasma levels, *Psychol. Med.,* 2: 111-120, 1972.

1179. IMABAYASHI, K. and MATSUMURA, S., Four cases of idiopathic renal hematuria with abnormal electroencephalogram, *Jap. J. Clin. Urol.,* 27: 139-144, 1973.

1180. INABA, T. and BRIEN, J. F., Determination of the major urinary metabolite of diphenylhydantoin by high-performance liquid chromatography, *J. Chromatogr.,* 80: 161-165, 1973.

1181. IOSUB, S., BINGOL, N., and WASSERMAN, E., The pregnant epileptic and her offspring, *Pediat. Res.,* 7: 420, 1973.

1182. ISAACS, H. and FRERE, G., Syndrome of continuous muscle fibre activity. Histochemical, nerve terminal and end-plate study of two cases, *South African Medical Journal,* 48: 1601-7, 1974.

1183. ISSACS, H., Continuous muscle fibre activity in an Indian male with additional evidence of terminal *40* motor fiber abnormality, *J. Neurol. Neurosurg. Psychiat.,* 30: 126-133, 1967.

1184. JANZ, D. and SCHMIDT, D., Comparison of spectrophotometric and gas liquid chromatographic measurements of serum diphenylhydantoin concentrations in epileptic outpatients, *Epilepsy Abstracts,* 7: 268, 1974.

1185. JANZ, D. and SCHMIDT, D., Anti-epileptic drugs and failure of oral contraceptives, *Lancet,* 1113, 1974.

1186. JENKINS, D. and SPECTOR, R. G., The actions of folate and phenytoin on the rat heart *in vivo* and *in vitro,* *Biochem. Pharmacol.,* 22: 1813-1816, 1973.

1187. JENSEN, O. N. and OLESEN, O. V., Subnormal serum folate due to anticonvulsive therapy, *Arch. Neurol.,* 22: 181-182, 1970.

1188. JENSEN, R. A. and KATZUNG, B. G., Electrophysiological actions of diphenylhydantoin on rabbit atria: dependence on stimulation frequency, potassium and sodium, *Circ. Res.,* 26: 17-27, 1970.

1189. JONAS, A. D., Diphenylhydantoin and the treatment of anxiety, *Amer. J. Psychiat.,* 126: 163, 1969. *13*

1190. JONES, G. L. and KEMP, J. W., Characteristics of the hydrogen bonding interactions of diphenylhydantoin with nucleic acids and their components, *Fed. Proc.,* 31: 570, 1972.

1191. JOVANOVIC, T., Experiences in the treatment of psychoses occurring concomitantly with epilepsy, *Neuropsihiatrija,* 20: 173-183, 1972.

1192. JOYNT, R. J. and GREEN, D., Tonic seizures as a manifestation of multiple sclerosis, *Arch. Neurol.,* 6: 293- *46* 299, 1962.

1193. JUBIZ, W. and Rallison, M. L., Diphenylhydantoin treatment of glycogen storage diseases, *Arch. Intern.* *50* *Med.,* 134: 418-421, 1974.

1194. JUBIZ, W., LEVINSON, R. A., MEIKLE, A. W., WEST, C. D., and TYLER, F. H., Absorption and conjugation of metyrapone during diphenylhydantoin therapy: mechanism of the abnormal response to oral metyrapone, *Endocrinology*, 86: 328-331, 1970.

1195. JUBIZ, W., MEIKLE, A. W., LEVINSON, R. A., MIZUTANI, S., WEST, C. D., and TYLER, F. H., Effect of diphenylhydantoin on the metabolism of dexamethasone, *New Eng. J. Med.*, 283: 11-14, 1970.

1196. JULIEN, R. M. and HALPERN, L. M., Cerebellar action of diphenylhydantoin on penicillin-induced cerebral cortical epileptic foci, *Fed. Proc.*, 29: Abstract 784, 1970.

1197. JULIEN, R. M. and HALPERN, L. M., Stabilization of excitable membrane by chronic administration of diphenylhydantoin, *J. Pharmacol. Exp. Ther.*, 175: 206-212, 1970.   *59*

1198. JULIEN, R. M. and HALPERN, L. M., Diphenylhydantoin: evidence for a central action, *Life Sci.*, 10: 575-582, 1971.   *60*

1199. JULIEN, R. M. and HALPERN, L. M., Effects of diphenylhydantoin and other antiepileptic drugs on epileptiform activity and Purkinje cell discharge rates, *Epilepsy Abstracts*, 5: 236, 1972.

1200. JUNG, S. S., CHEN, K. M., and BRODY, J. A., Paroxysmal choreoathetosis: report of Chinese cases, *Neurology*, 23: 749-755, 1973.   *44*

1201. JUS, K., JUS, A., GAUTIER, J., VILLENEUVE, A., PIRES, P., PINEAU, R. and VILLENEUVE, R., Studies on the action of certain pharmacological agents on tardive dyskinesia and on the rabbit syndrome, *Int. J. Clin. Pharmacol.*, 9: 138-145, 1974.

1202. KALMAN, P., NANASSY, A., and CSAPO, G., Diphenylhydantoin treatment of atrial tachycardia with heart block, *Z. Kardiologie*, 62: 75-79, 1972.

1203. KANZAWA, F., HOSHI, A., and KURETANI, K., Relationship between antitumor activity and chemical structure in psychotropic agents, *Gann*, 61: 529-534, 1970.

1204. KAPLAN, R., BLUME, S., ROSENBERG, S., PITRELLI, J., and TURNER, W. J., Phenytoin, metronidazole and multivitamins in the treatment of alcoholism, *Quart. J. Stud. Alcohol.*, 33: 97-104, 1972.

1205. KASAI, S. and YOSHIZUMI, T., Effect of diphenylhydantoin sodium on the proliferation of cultured cells *in vitro*, *Bull. Tokyo Dent. Coll.*, 12: 223-234, 1971.

1206. KATER, R. M. H., ROGGIN, G., Tobon, F., Zieve, P., and IBER, F. L., Increased rate of clearance of drugs from the circulation of alcoholics, *Amer. J. Med. Sci.*, 258: 35-39, 1969.

1207. KATER, R. M. H., TOBON, F., ZEIVE, P. D., ROGGIN, G. M., and IBER, F. L., Heavy drinking accelerates drugs' breakdown in liver, *JAMA*, 206: 1709, 1968.

1208. KATO, R., CHIESARA, E., and VASSANELLI, P., Increased activity of microsomal strychnine-metabolizing enzyme induced by phenobarbital and other drugs, *Biochem. Pharmacol.*, 11: 913-922, 1962.   *87*

1209. KAUFMANN, G. and HAUSER, K., Experience with diphenylhydantoin (antisacer) in the treatment of cardiac arrhythmias, *Schweiz. Med. Wschr.*, 98: 1223-1226, 1968.   *86*

1210. KAUFMANN, G. and WEBER-EGGENBERGER, S., Hemodynamic changes due to diphenylhydantoin in digitalized cardiac patients, *Schweiz. Med. Wschr.*, 100: 2164-2168, 1970.

1211. KAZAMATSURI, H., Elevated serum alkaline phosphatase levels in epilepsy during diphenylhydantoin therapy, *New Eng. J. Med.*, 283: 1411-1412, 1970.

1212. KAZAMATSURI, H., Elevated serum alkaline phosphatase levels in the epileptic patients with diphenylhydantoin, *Folia Psychiat. Neurol. Jap.*, 24: 181-189, 1970.

1213. KELTNER, J. L., BECKER, B., GAY, A. J., and PODOS, S. M., Effect of diphenylhydantoin in ischemic optic neuritis, *Trans. Amer. Ophthal. Soc.*, 70: 113-130, 1972.

1214. KEMP, G. L., Treatment of ventricular ectopic rhythms with diphenylhydantoin, *J. Amer. Geriat. Soc.*, 20: 265-267, 1972.   *25*

1215. KEMP, J. W. and WOODBURY, D. M., Subcellular distribution of 4-^{14}C-diphenylhydantoin in rat brain, *J. Pharmacol. Exp. Ther.*, 177: 342-349, 1971.   *92*

1216. KENNEDY, C., ANDERSON, W., and SOKOLOFF, L., Cerebral blood flow in epileptic children during the interseizure period, *Neurology*, 8: 100-105, 1958.   *30*

1217. KENNEDY, C., GRAVE, G. D., JEHLE, J. W., and KUPFERBERG, H. J., The effect of diphenylhydantoin on local cerebral blood flow, *Neurology*, 22: 451-452, 1972.

REFERENCES

1218. KESSLER, K. M., Individualization of dosage of antiarrhythmic drugs, *Medical Clinics of North America*, 58: 1019-26, 1974.

1219. KETEL, W. B. and HUGHES, J. R., Toxic encephalopathy with seizures secondary to ingestion of composition C-4, *Neurology*, 22: 871-876, 1972.

1220. KIZER, J. S., VARGAS-CORDON, M., BRENDEL, K., and BRESSLER, R., The *in vitro* inhibition of insulin secretion by diphenylhydantoin, *J. Clin. Invest.*, 49: 1942-1948, 1970.   *82*

1221. KLEINFELD, M. and STEIN, E., Effects of diphenylhydantoin on action potentials of canine Purkinje and ventricular fibers, *Circulation*, 38: 116, 1968.   *59*

1222. KNOPP, R. H., SHEININ, J. C., and FREINKEL, N., Diphenylhydantoin and an insulin-secreting islet adenoma, *Arch. Intern. Med.*, 130: 904-908, 1972.   *82*

1223. KOBAYASHI, I., YAMASHITA, Y., and YAMAZAKI, H., Onset of systemic lupus erythematosus during the long-term administration of diphenylhydantoin, *Nippon Naika Gakkai Zasshi*, 60: 851-854, 1971.

1224. KOCH-WESER, J., Antiarrhythmic prophylaxis in ambulatory patients with coronary heart disease, *Arch. Intern. Med.*, 129: 763-772, 1972.   *25*

1225. KOCH, A., HIGGINS, R., SANDE, M., TIERNEY, J., and TULIN, R., Enhancement of renal Na+ transport by Dilantin, *Physiologist*, 5: 168, 1962.   *63*

1226. KOCH, H. U., KRAFT, D., VON HERRATH, D., and SCHAEFER, K., Influence of diphenylhydantoin and phenobarbital on intestinal calcium transport in the rat, *Epilepsy Abstracts*, 6: 109, 1973.

1227. KOOTSTRA, A. and WOODHOUSE, S. P., The effect of diphenylhydantoin on the Na+-K+-stimulated ouabain-inhibited ATPase, *Proceedings of the University of Otago Medical School*, 52: 6-7, 1974.

1228. KOPPE, J. G., BOSMAN, W., OPPERS, V. M., SPAANS, F., and KLOOSTERMAN, G. J., Epilepsy and congenital anomalies, *Ned. T. Geneesk.*, 117: 220-224, 1973. (cf. Loughnan, et al., Lancet, 70, 1973.)

1229. KORMENDY, C. G. and BENDER, A. D., Experimental modification of the chemistry and biology of the aging process, *J. Pharm. Sci.*, 60: 167-180, 1971.

1230. KOSKI, C. L., RIFENBERICK, D. H., and MAX, S. R., Energy metabolism in steroid atrophy, *Neurology*, 4: 352, 1974.

1231. KOSTOV, K. G., TACHEV, A. M. and NASTEV, G. T., The problem of pseudomyotonia (Isaac's syndrome), *Zh. Nevropatol. Psikhiatr. Korsakov*, 73: 825-829, 1973.   *42*

1232. KRASNER, J., Drug-protein interaction, *Pediat. Clin. N. Amer.*, 19: 51-63, 1972.

1233. KRASNER, J., GIACOIA, G. P., and YAFFE, S. J., Drug protein binding in the newborn infant, *Pediat. Res.*, 7: 317, 1973.

1234. KRELL, R. D. and GOLDBERG, A. M., Effect of diphenylhydantoin and ethanol feeding on the synthesis of rat liver folates from exogenous pteroylglutamate (^{3}H), *Epilepsy Abstracts*, 7: 195, 1974.

1235. KRIKLER, D. M., A fresh look at cardiac arrhythmias, *Lancet*, 1034-1037, 1974.

1236. KRSIAK, M. and STEINBERG, H., Psychopharmacological aspects of aggression: a review of the literature and some new experiments, *J. Psychosom. Res.*, 13: 243-252, 1969.

1237. KRUGER, G., Effect of Dilantin in mice. 1. Changes in lymphoreticular tissue after acute exposure, *Virshows Arch.* (Path. Anat.), 349: 297-311, 1970. (*cf.* Juhasz, et al., *Acta Morphol. Acad. Sci. Hung.*, 18: 147, 1970.)

1238. KRUPIN, T., PODOS, S. M., and BECKER, B., Effect of diphenylhydantoin on dexamethasone suppression of plasma coritsol in primary open-angle glaucoma, *Amer. J. Ophthal.*, 71: 997-1002, 1971.

1239. KUIPER, J. J., Lymphocytic thyroiditis possibly induced by diphenylhydantoin, *JAMA*, 210: 2370-2372, 1969.

1240. KUNTZMAN, R. and SOUTHERN, A. L., The effects of CNS active drugs on the metabolism of steroids in man, *Adv. Biochem. Psychopharmacol.*, 1: 205-217, 1969.   *80*

1241. KUPFERBERG, H. J., Quantitative estimation of diphenylhydantoin, primidone and phenobarbital in plasma by gas-liquid chromatography, *Clin. Chim. Acta*, 29: 283-288, 1970.

1242. KUROIWA, Y. and ARAKI, S., Lhermitte's sign and reflex tonic spasm in demyelinating diseases with special reference to their localizing value, *Kyushu J. Med. Sci.*, 14: 29-38, 1963.

1243. Kuroiwa, Y. and Shibasaki, H., Painful tonic seizures in multiple sclerosis—treatment with diphenylhy- *46* dantoin and carbamazepine, *Folia. Psychiat. Neurol. Jap.*, 22: 107-119, 1968.

1244. Kutt, H. and Fouts, J. R., Diphenylhydantoin metabolism by rat liver microsomes and some of the effects of drug or chemical pretreatment on diphenylhydantoin metabolism by rat liver microsomal preparations, *J. Pharmacol. Exp. Ther.*, 176: 11-26, 1970.

1245. Kutt, H. and Penry, J. K., Usefulness of blood levels of antiepileptic drugs, *Arch. Neurol.*, 31: 283-288, 1974.

1246. Kutt, H. and Verebely, K., Metabolism of diphenylhydantoin by rat liver microsomes, *Biochem. Pharmacol.*, 19: 675-686, 1970.

1247. Kutt, H., Biochemical and genetic factors regulating Dilantin metabolism in man, *Ann. N. Y. Acad. Sci.*, 179: 704-722, 1971.

1248. Kutt, H., Diphenylhydantoin interactions with other drugs in man, *Antiepileptic Drugs*, 169-180, Woodbury, D. M., Penry, J. K., and Schmidt, R. P., Eds., Raven Press, New York, 1972. (*cf.* Evans, et al., *Lancet*, 517, 1970.)

1249. Kutt, H., Diphenylhydantoin relation of plasma levels to clinical control, *Antiepileptic Drugs*, 211-218, Woodbury, D. M., Penry, J. K., and Schmidt, R. P., Eds., Raven Press, New York, 1972.

1250. Kutt, H., Haynes, J., Verebely, K., and McDowell, F., The effect of phenobarbital on plasma diphenylhydantoin level and metabolism in man and rat liver microsomes, *Epilepsy Abstracts*, 3: 4, 1970.

1251. Kutt, H., Waters, L., and Fouts, J. R., Diphenylhydantoin-induced difference spectra with rat-liver microsomes, *Chem. Biol. Interactions*, 2: 195-202, 1970.

1252. Kutt, H., Waters, L., and Fouts, J. R., The effects of some stimulators (inducers) of hepatic microsomal drug-metabolizing enzyme activity on substrate-induced difference spectra in rat liver microsomes, *J. Pharmacol. Exp. Ther.*, 179: 101-113, 1971.

1253. Kwalick, D. S., Anticonvulsants and DDT residues, *JAMA*, 215: 120-121, 1971. *85*

1254. Kyosola, K., Abdominal epilepsy, *Ann. Chir. Gyanaec. Fenn.*, 62: 101-103, 1973.

1255. Lamprecht, F., Epilepsy and schizophrenia: a neurochemical bridge, *Epilepsy Abstracts*, 7: 190, 1974.

1256. Landolt, A. M., Treatment of acute post-operative inappropriate antidiuretic hormone secretion with *81* diphenylhydantoin, *Acta Endocr.*, 76: 625-628, 1974.

1257. Larsen, P. R., Atkinson, A. J., Wellman, H. N., and Goldsmith, R. E., Effect of diphenylhydantoin on thyroxine metabolism in man, *J. Clin. Invest.*, 49: 1266-1279, 1970.

1258. Lascelles, P. T., Kocen, R. S., and Reynolds, E. H., The distribution of plasma phenytoin levels in epileptic patients, *J. Neurol. Neurosurg. Psychiat.*, 33: 501-505, 1970.

1259. Lasser, R. P., Management of arrhythmia, *New York J. Med.*, 73: 1775-1777, 1973.

1260. Latham, A. N., Millbank, L., Richens, A., and Rowe, D. J. F., Liver enzyme induction by anticonvulsant drugs, and its relationship to disturbed calcium and folic acid metabolism, *J. Clin. Pharmacol.*, 13: 337-342, 1973.

1261. Lawrence, T., Antiarrhythmic drugs, *Topics on Medicinal Chemistry*, 3: 360-363, Wiley-Interscience, New York, 1970.

1262. Lee, S. I. and Bass, N. H., Microassay of diphenylhydantoin: blood and regional brain concentrations in rats during acute intoxication, *Neurology*, 20: 115-124, 1970.

1263. Lefebvre, E. B., Haining, R. G., and Labbe, R. F., Coarse facies, calvarial thickening and hyperphosphatasia associated with long-term anticonvulsant therapy, *New Eng. J. Med.*, 286: 1301-1302, 1972. (*cf.* Falcone and Davidson, *Lancet*, 2: 1112, 1973, Griscom, *New Eng. J. Med.*, 287: 722, 1972, Lefebvre, et al., Nellhaus and Poskanzer, *ibid.*)

1264. Lesbre, J. P., Cathala, B., Salvador, M., Florio, R., Lescure, F., and Meriel, P., Diphenylhydantoin *25* and digitalis toxicity, *Arch. Mal. Coeur.*, 62: 412-437, 1969.

1265. Lesne, M., Sturbois, X. and Wilmotte, L., Modifications by diphenylhydantoin of the pharmacokinetic of digitoxin in the rat, *J. Pharmacol.*, 5: 75-86, 1974.

1266. Letteri, J. M., Mellk, H., Louis, S., Kutt, H., Durante, P., and Glazko, A., Diphenylhydantoin metabolism in uremia, *New Eng. J. Med.*, 285: 648-652, 1971.

REFERENCES

—————————————————————————————— *Page*

1267. LeVan, H., Gordon, P., and Stefani, S., Enhancement of radioresistance in mice treated with diphenylhydantoin, *J. Pharm. Sci.*, 59: 1178-1179, 1970.

1268. LeVan, H., Gordon, P., and Stefani, S., Effect of diphenylhydantoin on survival and morphology of Ehrlich ascites tumor mice, *Oncology*, 26: 25-32, 1972.

1269. Levin, S. R., Booker, J., Smith, D. F., and Grodsky, G. M., Inhibition of insulin secretion by diphenylhydantoin in the isolated perfused pancreas, *J. Clin. Endocr.*, 300: 400-401, 1970.   *82*

1270. Levin, S. R., Charles, M. A., O'Connor, M., and Grodsky, G. M., Use of diphenylhydantoin and diazoxide to investigate insulin secretory mechanisms, *Presented at the 8th Congress of International Diabetes Federation*, Brussels, Belgium, 1973.

1271. Levin, S. R., Charles, M. A., O'Connor, M., Hagura, R., Smith, D., and Grodsky, G. M., Comparative effects of diphenylhydantoin (DPH) and diazoxide (DZ) upon biphasic insulin secretion from the isolated, perfused rat pancreas, with computerized correlation of biologic responses, *Presented at the International Diabetes Congress in Belgium*, 1973.

1272. Levin, S. R., Grodsky, G., Hagura, R., Smith, D., Licko, V., and Forsham, P., Comparison of effects of   *83* diphenylhydantoin and diazoxide on insulin secretion in the isolated perfused rat pancreas, using computerized correlation of experimental data, *Clin. Res.*, 19: 375, 1971.

1273. Levin, S. R., Grodsky, G. M., Hagura, R., and Smith, D., Comparison of the inhibitory effects of   *83* diphenylhydantoin and diazoxide upon insulin secretion from the isolated perfused pancreas, *Diabetes*, 21: 856-862, 1972. (*cf.* Goldberg, *Diabetes*, 18: 101, 1969.)

1274. Levin, S. R., Reed, J. W., Ching, K. N., Davis, J. W., and Blum, R., Inhibition of insulin secretion after   *83* diphenylhydantoin (DPH) in diabetes and in obesity, *Clin. Res.*, 20: 178, 1972.

1275. Levin, S. R., Reed, J. W., Ching, K. N., Davis, J. W., Blum, M. R., and Forsham, P. H., Diphenylhydantoin: its use in detecting early insulin secretory defects in patients with mild glucose intolerance, *Diabetes*, 22: 194-201, 1973.

1276. Levine, M. C., Reactions to anticonvulsants, *New Eng. J. Med.*, 286: 1217, 1972.

1277. Levitt, B., Raines, A., Sohn, Y. J., Standaert, F. G., and Hirshfeld, J. W., The nervous system as a site   *86* of action for digitalis and antiarrhythmic drugs, *Mt. Sinai Med. J.*, 37: 227-240, 1970.

1278. Levitt, M., Nixon, P. F., Pincus, J. H., and Bertino, J. R., Transport characteristics of folates in cerebrospinal fluid; a study utilizing doubly labeled 5-methyltetrahydrofolate and 5-formyltetrahydrofolate, *J. Clin. Invest.*, 50: 1301-1308, 1971.

1279. Levo, Y., The protective effect of hydantoin treatment on carcinogenesis, *Naunyn-Schmiedeberg's Arch.*   *91* *Pharmacol.*, 285: 29-30, 1974.

1280. Levy, J. A., Wittig, E. O., Ferraz, E. C. F., Scleroderma associated with continuous electro-muscular   *41* activity, *Arq. Neuro-Psiquiat*, 23: 283-287, 1965.

1281. Levy, R. H. and Smith, G. H., Dosage regimens of antiarrhythmics, Part 1: Pharmacokinetic properties, *Amer. J. Hosp. Pharm.*, 30: 398-404, 1973.

1282. Lew, G. M., Increased hypothalamic norepinephrine in genetically hypertensive rats following administration of diphenylhydantoin, *Proc. Soc. Exp. Biol. Med.*, 148: 30-32, 1975.   *75*

1283. Lewin, E. and Bleck, V., The effect of diphenylhydantoin administration on sodium-potassium-activated ATPase in cortex, *Neurology*, 21: 647-651, 1971.

1284. Lewin, E. and Bleck, V., The effect of diphenylhydantoin administration on cortex potassium-activated phosphatase, *Neurology*, 21: 417-418, 1971.

1285. Lewin, E., Charles, G., and McCrimmon, A., Discharging cortical lesions produced by freezing—the effect of anticonvulsants on sodium-potassium-activated ATPase, sodium, and potassium in cortex, *Neurology*, 19: 565-569, 1969.

1286. Lien, E. J. and Gudauskas, G. A., Structure side-effect sorting of drugs—I: Extrapyramidal syndrome, *J. Pharm. Sci.*, 62: 645-647, 1973.

1287. Lifshitz, F. and Maclaren, N. K., Vitamin D-dependent rickets in institutionalized, mentally retarded childred receiving long-term anticonvulsant therapy, *J. Pediat.*, 83: 612-620, 1973.

1288. LIGHTFOOT, R. W., JR., and CHRISTIAN, C. L., Serum protein binding of thyroxine and diphenylhydantoin, *J. Clin. Endocr.*, 26: 305-308, 1966.

1289. LINDE, L. M., TURNER, S. W., and AWA, S., Present status and treatment of paroxysmal supraventricular tachycardia, *Pediatrics*, 50: 127-130, 1972.   *29*

1290. LIPICKY, R. J., GILBERT, D. L., and STILLMAN, I. M., The effects of diphenylhydantoin on voltage-dependent currents of the squid axon, *Fed. Proc.*, 30: Abstract 65, 1971.

1291. LIPICKY, R. J., GILBERT, D. L., and STILLMAN, I. M., Diphenylhydantoin inhibition of sodium conductance in squid giant axon, *Proc. Nat. Acad. Sci.*, 69: 1758-1760, 1972.   *60*

1292. LISAK, R. P., LEBEAU, J., TUCKER, S. H., and ROWLAND, L. P., Hyperkalemic periodic paralysis and cardiac arrhythmia, *Neurology*, 22: 810-815, 1972.

1293. LIVINGSTON, S., Abdominal pain as a manifestation of epilepsy (abdominal epilepsy) in children, *J. Pediat.*, 38: 687-695, 1951.

1294. LIVINGSTON, S. and LIVINGSTON, H. L., Diphenylhydantoin gingival hyperplasia, *Amer. J. Dis. Child.*, 117: 265-270, 1969.

1295. LIVINGSTON, S. and PAULI, L. L., Diphenylhydantoin and blood dyscrasias, *JAMA*, 320: 211-212, 1974.

1296. LIVINGSTON, S., BERMAN, W., and PAULI, L. L., Anticonvulsant drugs and vitamin D metabolism, *JAMA*, 224: 1634-1635, 1973.

1297. LIVINGSTON, S., BERMAN, W., and PAULI, L. L., Anticonvulsant drugs and vitamin D metabolism, *JAMA*, 226: 787, 1973.

1298. LIVINGSTON, S., BERMAN, W., and PAULI, L. L., Maternal epilepsy and abnormalities of the fetus and newborn, *Lancet*, 2: 1265, 1973.

1299. LOCKMAN, L. A., HUNNINGHAKE, D. B., KRIVIT, W., and DESNICK, R. J., Relief of pain of Fabry's disease by diphenylhydantoin, *Neurology*, 23: 871-875, 1973.   *36*

1300. LOCKMAN, L. A., KRIVIT, W., and DESNICK, R. J., Relief of the painful crises of Fabry's disease by diphenylhydantoin, *Neurology*, 21: 423, 1971.

1301. LOESER, J. D., Neuralgia, *Postgrad. Med.*, 53: 207-210, 1973.

1302. LOHRENZ, J. G., LEVY, L., and DAVIS, J. F., Schizophrenia or epilepsy? A problem in differential diagnosis, *Compr. Psychiat.*, 3: 54-62, 1962.

1303. LONGSHAW, R. N., Inhibition of hepatic drug metabolism, *Drug Intelligence and Clinical Pharmacy*, 7: 263-270, 1973.

1304. LOOKER, A. and CONNERS, C. K., Diphenylhydantoin in children with severe temper tantrums, *Arch. Gen.   13 Psychiat.*, 23: 80-89, 1970.

1305. LOONG, S. C. and ONG, Y. Y., Paroxysmal kinesigenic choreoathetosia, *J. Neurol. Neurosurg. Psychiat.*,   *44* 36: 921-924, 1973.

1306. LOTTI, V. J., TORCHIANA, M. L., and PORTER, C. C., Investigations on the action and mechanism of action   *91* of diphenylhydantoin as an antagonist of tetrabenazine and reserpine, *Arch. Int. Pharmacodyn.*, 203: 107-116, 1973.

1307. LOTTO, A., SANNA, G. P., BOSSI, M., and LOMANTO, B., New therapeutic aspects of ventricular arrhythmias, *Cardiol. Prat.*, 22: 1-15, 1971.

1308. LOUIS, S., KUTT, H., and McDOWELL, F., Modification of experimental seizures and anticonvulsant efficacy by peripheral stimulation, *Neurology*, 21: 329-336, 1971.

1309. LOVELL, R. R. H., MITCHELL, M. E., PRINEAS, R. J., SLOMAN, J. G., VAJDA, F. J., PITT, A., HABERSBERGER, P., ROSENBAUM, M., NESTEL, P. J., GOODMAN, H. T, and SOWRY, G. S. C., Phenytoin after recovery from myocardial infarction—controlled trial in 568 patients, *Lancet*, 1055-1057, 1971.

1310. LOWE, C. R., Congenital malformations among infants born to epileptic women, *Lancet*, 9-10, 1973. (*cf.* Marsh and Fraser, *Teratology*, 7: A-23, 1973.)

1311. LOWN, B., TEMTE, J. V. and ARTER, W. J., Ventricular tachyarrhythmias—clinical aspects, *Circulation*, 47: 1364-1381, 1973.

1312. LUCCHESI, B. R., The pharmacology and clinical uses of antiarrhythmic drugs, *U. Michigan Med. Cent. J.*, 37: 61-73, 1971.

REFERENCES

_____ *Page*

1313. LUDTKE, A. H., AUTENRIETH, G., and DANKERT, D., On the effects of diphenylhydantoin, potassium-magnesium-asparaginate, insulin and female sex hormones on the hypothermic fibrillation threshold of the guinea-pig heart, *Arzneimittelforschung*, 20: 1554-1557, 1970.

1314. LUND, L., BERLIN, A., and LUNDE, K. M., Plasma protein binding of diphenylhydantoin in patients with epilepsy, *Clin. Pharmacol. Ther.*, 13: 196-200, 1972.

1315. LUNDE, K. M., Plasma protein binding of diphenylhydantoin in man, *Acta Pharmacol.*, 29: 152-155, 1971.

1316. LUNDE, K. M., RANE, A., YAFFE, S. J., LUND, L., and SJOQVIST, F., Plasma protein binding of diphenylhydantoin in man, *Clin. Pharmacol. Ther.*, 11: 846-855, 1970.

1317. LUND, L., LUNDE, P. K., RANE, A., BORGA, O. and SJOQVIST, F., Plasma protein binding, plasma concentrations, and effects of diphenylhydantoin in man, *Ann. N.Y. Acad. Sci.*, 179: 723-728, 1972.

1318. LUSSIER-LAZAROFF, J. and FLETCHER, B. D., Rickets and anticonvulsant therapy in children: a roentgenologic investigation, *J. Canad. Assn. Radiol.*, 22: 144-147, 1971.

1319. LUTZ, E. G., Add vitamins to DPH, urges doctor, *National Spokesman*, 6: 7, 1973.

1320. LUTZ, E. G., On vitamins and anticonvulsants, *Medical World News*, 3, 1973.

1321. MACE, J., and SCHNEIDER, S., Diphenylhydantoin and rickets, *Lancet*, 1119, 1973.

1322. MACGEE, J., The rapid determination of diphenylhydantoin in blood plasma by gas-liquid chromatography, *Med. Res. Lab., V.A. Hosp. and Dept. Bio. Chem. and Exp. Med.*, Cincinnati, Ohio, 1970.

1323. MACKINNEY, A. A. and BOOKER, H. E., Diphenylhydantoin effects on human lymphocytes *in vitro* and *in vivo*, *Arch. Intern. Med.*, 129: 988-992, 1972.

1324. MACKINNEY, A. A. and VYAS, R., Diphenylhydantoin-induced inhibition of nucleic acid synthesis in cultured human lymphocytes, *Proc. Soc. Exp. Biol. Med.*, 141: 89-92, 1972.

1325. MACKINNEY, A. A. and VYAS, R., The assay of diphenylhydantoin effects on growing human lymphocytes, *J. Pharmacol. Exp. Ther.*, 186: 37-43, 1973.

1326. MACLAREN, N. and LIFSHITZ, F., Vitamin D-dependency rickets in institutionalized, mentally retarded children on long term anticonvulsant therapy. II. The response to 25-hydroxycholecalciferol and to vitamin D, *Pediat. Res.*, 7: 914-922, 1973.

1327. MADSEN, S. N., HANSEN, J. M. and DECKERT, T., Intravenous glucose tolerance during treatment with phenytoin, *Acta Neurol. Scand.*, 50: 257-260, 1974.   *83*

1328. MALETZKY, B. M. and KLOTTER, J., Episodic dyscontrol: A controlled replication, *Dis. Nerv. Syst.*, 35: 175-179, 1974.   *15*

1329. MALETZKY, B. M., Treatable violence, *Med. Times*, 100: 74-79, 1972.   *15*

1330. MALHERBE, C., BURRILL, K. C., LEVIN, S. R., KARAM, J. H., and FORSHAM, P. H., Effect of diphenylhydantoin on insulin secretion in man, *New Eng. J. Med.*, 286: 339-342, 1972.

1331. MARKKANEN, T., HIMANEN, P., PAJULA, R. L., and MOLNAR, G., Binding of folic acid to serum proteins, *Acta Haemat.*, 50: 284-292, 1973.

1332. MARKKANEN, T., PELTOLA, O., HIMANEN, P. and RIEKKINEN, P., Metabolites of diphenylhydantoin in human plasma inhibits the pentose phosphate pathway of leukocytes, *Pharmacology*, 6: 216-222, 1971.

1333. MARTIN, C. M., Reliability in product performance in an innovative environment, The Economics of Drug Innovation, 63-82, Cooper, J. D., Ed., *The Proceedings of the First Seminar of Economics of Pharmaceutical Innovation*, 1969.

1334. MARTIN, W. and RICKERS, J., Cholestatic hepatosis induced by diphenylhydantoin. Case report and review of literature, *Wien. Klin. Wschr.*, 84: 41-45, 1972.

1335. MASON, D. T., AMSTERDAM, E. A., MASSUMI, R. A. and ZELIS, R., Recent advances in antiarrhythmic drugs: clinical pharmacology and therapeutics, *The Acute Cardiac Emergencey—Diagnosis and Management*, 95-123, Eliot, R. S., Ed., Futura Publishing, Mount Kisco, New York, 1972.

1336. MASON, D. T., DeMARIA, A. N., AMSTERDAM, E. A., ZELIS, R., and MASSUMI, R. A., Antiarrhythmic agents. II: Therapeutic consideration, *Drugs*, 5: 292-317, 1973.

1337. MASON, D. T., DeMARIA, A. N., AMSTERDAM, E. A., ZELIS, R., and MASSUMI, R. A., Antiarrhythmic agents. I: Mechanisms of action and clinical pharmacology, *Drugs*, 5: 261-291, 1973.

1338. MASON, D. T., SPANN, J. F., JR., ZELIS, R., and AMSTERDAM, E. A., Evolving concepts in the clinical pharmacology and therapeutic uses of the antiarrhythmic drugs, *Cardiovascular Therapy, The Art and the Science*, 122-137, Russek, H. I. and Zohman, B. L., Eds., The Williams & Wilkins, Co., Baltimore, 1971.

1339. MATHUR, K. S., WAHAL, P. K., SETH, H. C., and HAZRA, D. K., Diphenylhydantoin sodium in cardiac arrhythmias, *J. Indian Med. Assoc.*, 57: 256-258, 1971.   25

1340. MATSUZAKI, M. and KILLAM, K. F., Alterations in conditional behavioral and electrographic responses to interrupted visual stimuli following repeated doses of diphenylhydantoin, *Fed. Proc.*, 30: Abstract 483, 1971.

1341. MATTES, L. M., SPRITZER, R. C., NEVINS, M. A., WEISENSEEL, A. C., DONOSO, E., and FRIEDBURG, C. K., The cardiovascular effects of diphenylhydantoin in patients with cardiac pacemakers, *Circulation*, 37-38 (Suppl. 6): 135, 1968.

1342. MATTHEWS, W. B., Tonic seizures in disseminated sclerosis, *Brain*, 81: 193-206, 1958.   46

1343. MATTHEWS, W. D. and CONNOR, J. D., Effects of diphenylhydantoin on interhippocampal evoked responses, *Pharmacologist*, 16: 228, 1974.   62

1344. MATTSON, R. H., GALLAGHER, B. B., REYNOLDS, E. H., and GLASS, D., Folate therapy in epilepsy, *Arch. Neurol.*, 29: 78-81, 1973.

1345. McALLISTER, R. G., JR., The possible role of antiarrhythmic drugs in the prevention of sudden death, *Heart and Lung*, 2: 857-861, 1973.

1346. McCABE, B. F., Chronic burning tongue syndrome, *Ann. Otol. Rhinol. Laryngol*, 83: 264, 1974.

1347. McCABE, W. S. and HABOVICK, J. A., Thorazine as an epileptogenic agent, *Amer. J. Psychiat.*, 120: 595-597, 1963.

1348. McILVANIE, S. K., Phenytoin and depression of immunological function, *Lancet*, 323, February, 1972.

1349. McQUEEN, E. G., OWEN, D., and FERRY, D. G., Effect of phenytoin and other drugs in reducing serum DDT levels, *New Zeal. Med. J.*, 75: 208-211, 1972.   85

1350. MEADOW, S. R., Anticonvulsant drugs and congenital abnormalities, *Lancet*, 2: 1296, 1968.

1351. MEIKLE, W., JUBIZ, W., WEST, C. D., and TYLER, F. H., Effect of diphenylhydantoin (Dilantin) on the metyrapone test demonstrated by a new assay for plasma metyrapone, *Clin. Res.*, 17: 107, 1969.   81

1352. MELIKIAN, V., EDDY, J. D., and PATON, A., The stimulant effect of drugs on indocyanine green clearance by the liver, *Gut*, 13: 755-758, 1972.

1353. MENDELSON, J. H., Biologic concomitants of alcoholism, *New Eng. J. Med.*, 283: 24-32, 1970.

1354. MENNEAR, J. H. and GOSSEL, T. A., Inhibitory effect of diphenylhydantoin on the diabetogenic action of alloxan in the mouse, *Diabetes*, 21: 80-83, 1972.   85

1355. MENNEAR, J. H. and GOSSEL, T. A., Interactions between diphenylhydantoin and tolbutamide in mice, *Toxic. Appl. Pharmacol.*, 24: 309-316, 1973.   84

1356. MEYER, J. G., The teratological effects of anticonvulsants and the effects on pregnancy and birth, *Europ. Neurol.*, 10: 179-190, 1973.

1357. MEYER, J. S., BINNS, P. M., ERICSSON, A. D., and VULPE, M., Sphenopalatine ganglionectomy for cluster headache, *Arch. Otolaryng.*, 92: 475-484, 1970.

1358. MICHELL, A. R., The effect of diphenylhydantoin on sodium appetite in rats, *J. Physiol.*, 237: 53-55, 1973.

1359. MICK, B. A., Diphenylhydantoin and intermittent edema, *JAMA*, 225: 1533, 1973.   53

1360. MILEY, C. E. and FORSTER, F. M., Paroxysmal signs and symptoms in multiple sclerosis, *Neurology*, 24: 458-461, 1974.

1361. MILLICHAP, J. G., Clinical efficacy and usage of anticonvulsants, *Chemical Modulation of Brain Function*, 199-205, Sabelli, H. C., Ed., Raven Press, New York, 1973.

1362. MILLICHAP, J. G., Drugs in management of minimal brain dysfunction, *Ann. N. Y. Acad. Sci.*, 205: 321-334, 1973.

1363. MILLICHAP, J. G., Efficacy, therapeutic regimens of drugs to control hyperkinesis in children with minimal brain dysfunction reported from trials, *Drug Res. Rep.*, 15: S5-S11, 1972.

REFERENCES

—— *Page*

1364. MIRKIN, B. L. and WRIGHT, F., Drug interactions: effect of methylphenidate on the disposition of diphenylhydantoin in man, *Neurology*, 21: 1123-1128, 1971.

1365. MIRKIN, B. L., Diphenylhydantoin: placental transport, fetal localization, neonatal metabolism, and possible teratogenic effects, *J. Pediat.*, 78: 329-337, 1971.

1366. MIRKIN, B. L., Maternal and fetal distribution of drugs in pregnancy, *Clin. Pharmacol. Ther.*, 14: 643-647, 1973.

1367. MIRKIN, B. L., Placental transfer and neonatal elimination of diphenylhydantoin, *Amer. J. Obstet. Gynec.*, 109: 930-933, 1971.

1368. MITTLER, J. C. and GLICK, S. M., Radioimmunoassayable oxytocin release from isolated neural lobes: responses to ions and drugs, *Abstracts Fourth Int. Cong. Endocr.*, 47, June, 1972.   *81*

1369. MLADINICH, E. K., Diphenylhydantoin in the Wallenberg syndrome, *JAMA 230: 372-373*, 1974.   *38*

1370. MONSON, R. R., ROSENBERG, L., HARTZ, S. C., SHAPIRO, S., HEINONEN, O. P., and SLONE, D., Diphenylhydantoin and selected congenital malformations, *New Eng. J. Med.*, 289: 1050-1052, 1973.

1371. MORGAN, R. J., Scleroderma: treatment with diphenylhydantoin, *Cutis*, 8: 278-282, 1971.   *48*

1372. MOSS, A. J. and PATTON, R. D., Diphenylhydantoin, comparison of antiarrhythmic agents, and management of refractory arrhythmias, *Antiarrhythmic Agents*, 52-58, 101-115, Charles C. Thomas, Springfield, Ill., 1973.

1373. MOSS, G. and STEIN, A. A., Cerebral etiology of the shock lung syndrome: protective effect of diphenylhydantoin, *Personal Communication*, 1972.

1374. MOSS, G., Shock, cerebral hypoxia, and pulmonary vascular control: the centri-neurogenic etiology of the "respiratory distress syndrome", *Bull. N. Y. Acad. Med.*, 49: 689, 1973.   *67*

1375. MOUNTAIN, K. R., HIRSH, J., and GALLUS, A. S., Neonatal coagulation defect due to anticonvulsant drug treatment in pregnancy, *Lancet*, 1: 265-268, 1970. (*cf.* Davies, *Lancet*, 1: 413, 1970.)

1376. MOURAVIEFF-LESUISSE, F. and GIURGEA, C., Influence of electro-convulsive shock on the fixation of an experience at spinal level, *Arch. Int. Pharmacodyn.*, 183: 410-411, 1970.   *89*

1377. NABWANGU, J. F., Head injury, *E. Afr. Med. J.*, 49: 624-629, 1972.

1378. NARISAWA, K., HONDA, Y., and ARAKAWA, T., Effect of diphenylhydantoin administration on single carbon metabolism in folate deficient rats, *Tohoku, J. Exp. Med.*, 110: 359-365, 1973.

1379. NASELLO, A. G., MONTINI, E. E., and ASTRADA, C. A., Effect of veratrine, tetraethylammonium and diphenylhydantoin on potassium release by rat hippocampus, *Pharmacology*, 7: 89-95, 1972.   *64*

1380. NEGRI, S., An atypical case of Steinert's disease (myotonia dystrophica) in infancy, *Confin. Neurol.*, 33: 323-333, 1971.

1381. NEVILLE, B. G. R., The origin of infantile spasms: evidence from a case of hydranencephaly, *Epilepsy Abstracts*, 6: 179, 1973.

1382. NEWTOWN, R., Amitriptyline and imipramine poisoning in children, *Brit. Med. J.*, 2: 176, 1974.   *85*

1383. NIELSEN, T. and COTMAN, C., The binding of diphenylhydantoin to brain and subcellular fractions, *Europ. J. Pharmacol.*, 14: 344-350, 1971.   *93*

1384. NISWANDER, J. D. and WERTELECKI, W., Congenital malformation among offspring of epileptic women, *Lancet*, 1062, May, 1973.

1385. NOACH, E. L., VANREES, H. and DEWOLFF, F. A., Effects of Diphenylhydantoin (DPH) on absorptive processes in the rat jejunum, *Archives Internationales de Pharmacodynamie et de Therapie*, 206: 392-393, 1973.   *64*

1386. NORRIS, J. W. and PRATT, R. F., A controlled study of folic acid in epilepsy, *Neurology*, 21: 659-664, 1971.

1387. NUKI, K. and COOPER, S. H., The role of inflammation in the pathogenesis of gingival enlargement during the administration of diphenylhydantoin sodium in cats, *J. Periodont. Res.*, 7: 102-110, 1972.

1388. O'LEARY, J. A., FELDMAN, M., and SWITZER, H. E., Phenobarbital-Dilantin treatment of the intrauterine patient, *J. Reprod. Med.*, 5: 81-83, 1970.   *85*

1389. O'MALLEY, W. E., DENCKLA, M. B., and O'DOHERTY, D. S., Oral absorption of diphenylhydantoin as measured by gas liquid chromatography, *Epilepsy Abstracts*, 3: 230, 1970.

1390. O'REILLY, M. V. and MACDONALD, R. T., Efficacy of phenytoin in the management of ventricular *28*
arrhythmias induced by hypokalaemia, *Brit. Heart J.*, 35: 631-634, 1973.

1391. OATES, R. K. and TONGE, R. E., Phenytoin and the pseudolymphoma syndrome, *Med. J. Aust.*, 371-373,
1971.

1392. OBBENS, E. A., Experimental epilepsy induced by folate derivatives, *Epilepsy Abstracts*, 6: 221-222, 1973.

1393. ODAR-CEDERLOF, I. and BORGA, O., Kinetics of diphenylhydantoin in uraemic patients: consequences of
decreased plasma protein binding, *Europ. J. Clin. Pharmacol.*, 7: 31-37, 1974.

1394. OGE, V., Drug therapy in alcoholism, *Ill. Med. J.*, 139: 606-610, 1971.

1395. OLDS, M. E., Comparative effects of amphetamine, scopolamine, chlordiazepoxide, and diphenylhydantoin on operant and extinction behavior with brain stimulation and food reward, *Neuropharmacology*, 9: 519-532, 1970.

1396. OSORIO, C., JACKSON, D. J., GARTSIDE, J. M., and GOOLDEN, A. W. G., Effect of carbon dioxide and
diphenylhydantoin on the partition of triiodothyronine labelled with iodine-131 between the red cells
and plasma proteins, *Nature*, 196: 275-276, 1962.

1397. OVERALL, J. E., BROWN, D., WILLIAMS, J. D., and NEILL, L. T., Drug treatment of anxiety and depression
in detoxified alcoholic patients, *Arch. Gen. Psychiat.*, 29: 218-221, 1973.

1398. PAKSZYS, W. and DOMZAL, T., Ceruloplasmin stimulation test, *Epilepsy Abstracts*, 7: 107, 1974.

1399. PAKSZYS, W., Phenytoin, *Epilepsy Abstracts*, 6: 236, 1973.

1400. PARISI, A. F. and RAINES, A., Diphenylhydantoin suppression of repetitive activity generated in nerve *58*
endings, *Fed. Proc.*, Abstract 22: 390, 1963.

1401. PASHAYAN, H., PRUZANSKY, D., and PRUZANSKY, S., Are anticonvulsants teratogenic?, *Lancet*, 702-703,
1971.

1402. PATTON, R. D. and HELFANT, R. H., Atrial flutter with one-to-one conduction, *Dis. Chest*, 55: 250-251, *86*
1969.

1403. PAYEN, J., A study of changes in the gum during treatment with diphenylhydantoin sodium, *Rev.* *51*
Odonto-Stomatol., 19: 47-53, 1972.

1404. PELKONEN, R. and TASKINEN, M. R., Effect of diphenylhydantoin on plasma-insulin in insulinoma, *82*
Lancet, 604-605, 1973.

1405. PENTO, J. T., GLICK, S. M., and KAGAN, A., Diphenylhydantoin inhibition of glucagon- and calcium-
stimulated calcitonin release, *Fed. Proc.*, Abstract 31: 251, 1972.

1406. PENTO, J. T., GLICK, S. M., and KAGAN, A., Diphenylhydantoin inhibition of calcitonin secretion in the *77*
pig, *Endocrinology*, 92: 330-333, 1973.

1407. PENTTILA, O., NEUVONEN, P. J., AHO, K. and LEHTOVAARA, R., Interaction between doxycycline and some
antiepileptic drugs, *Brit. Med. J.*, 2: 470-472, 1974.

1408. PERSIJN, G. G. and VAN ZEBEN, W., Generalized lymphadenopathy caused by phenytoin in a six year old
child, *Epilepsy Abstracts*, 6: 236, 1973.

1409. PETER, J. B., A (Na+K) ATPase of sarcolemma from skeletal muscle, *Biochem. Biophys. Res. Commun.*,
40: 1362-1367, 1970.

1410. PETERS, B. H. and SAMAAN, N. A., Hyperglycemia with relative hypoinsulinemia in diphenylhydantoin
toxicity, *New Eng. J. Med.*, 281: 91-92, 1969.

1411. PETROSKI, D. and PATEL, A. N., Diphenylhydantoin for intractable hiccups, *Lancet*, 1: 739, 1974. *46*

1412. PEZCON, J. D. and GRANT, W. M., Sedatives, stimulants, and intraocular pressure in glaucoma, *Arch.*
Ophthal., 72: 177-188, 1964.

1413. PEZZIMENTI, J. F. and HAHN, A. L., Anicteric hepatitis induced by diphenylhydantoin, *Arch. Intern.*
Med., 125: 118-120, 1970.

1414. PHILLIPS, J. R. and ELDRIDGE, F. L., Respiratory myoclonus (Leeuwenhoek's disease), *New Eng. J. Med.*, *47*
289: 1390-1395, 1973.

1415. PINTO, A., SIMOPOULOS, A. M., McGEE, J. J., UHLENHUTH, E. W. and DeROSA, E. R., Enhanced ther- *16*
apeutic effects when DPH is added to phenothiazines in chronic schizophrenics, *(As Yet Unpublished)*
1974.

REFERENCES

── *Page*

1416. PINCUS, J. H. and LEE, S. H., Diphenylhydantoin and norepinephrine release, *Neurology*, 22: 410, 1972.

1417. PINCUS, J. H. and LEE, S. H., Diphenylhydantoin and calcium in relation to norepinephrine release from brain slices, *Arch. Neurol.*, 29: 239-244, 1973.   *77*

1418. PINCUS, J. H., Diphenylhydantoin and ion flux in lobster nerve, *Arch. Neurol.*, 26: 4-10, 1972.   *64*

1419. PINCUS, J. H., GROVE, I., MARINO, B. B. and GLASER, G. E., Studies on the mechanism of action of diphenylhydantoin, *Presented at the International Soc. Neurochem.*, September, 1969.   *67*

1420. PINKHAS, J., BEN-BASSAT, M., and DEVRIES, A., Death in anticonvulsant-induced megaloblastic anemia, *JAMA*, 224: 246, 1973.

1421. PODOS, S. M., BECKER, B., BEATY, C., and COOPER, D. G., Diphenylhydantoin and cortisol metabolism in glaucoma, *Amer. J. Ophthal.*, 74: 498-500, 1972.

1422. PODOS, S. M., Glaucoma, *Invest. Ophthal.*, 12: 3-4, 1973.

1423. POLEY, J. R. and BHATIA, M., Recurrent abdominal pain: recurrent controversy, *Pediatrics*, 52: 144-145, 1973.

1424. POLLEN, R. H., Cat-scratch encephalitis, *Neurology*, 18: 1031-1033, 1968.

1425. PORCIELLO, P. I. and ZANINI, S., Diphenylhydantoin: anti-arrhythmic drug, *Fracastoro*, 64: 114-135, 1971.

1426. PORCIELLO, P. I., ZANINI, S., and POPPI, A., Comparative considerations on two modern antiarrhythmic drugs: lidocaine and diphenylhydantoin, *G. Ital. Cardiol.* 2: 579-583, 1972.

1427. POSCHEL, B. P. H., A simple and specific screen for benzodiazepine-like drugs, *Psychopharmacologia*, 19: 193-198, 1971.

1428. POSTLETHWAITE, R. J. and PRICE, D. A., Amitriptyline and imipramine poisoning in children, *Brit. Med. J.*, 2: 504, 1974.   *85*

1429. PRESTON, T. A., YATES, J. D., and BRYMER, J. F., Three therapeutic approaches in tachycardia, *Geriatrics*, 28: 110-116, 1973.

1430. PRICE, D. A. and POSTLETHWAITE, J. R., Amitriptyline and imipramine poisoning in children, *Brit. Med. J.*, 1: 575, 1974.   *85*

1431. PRYLES, C. V., Livingston, S., and FORD, F. R., Familial paroxysmal choreoathetosis of Mount and Reback, *Pediatrics*, 9: 44-47, 1952.

1432. PURI, P. S., The effect of diphenylhydantoin sodium (Dilantin) on myocardial contractility and hemodynamics, *Amer. Heart J.*, 82: 62-68, 1971.

1433. PURO, D. G. and WOODWARD, D. J., Effects of diphenylhydantoin on activity of rat crebellar Purkinje cells, *Neuropharmacology*, 12: 433-440, 1973.

1434. QUIRET, J. C., BENS, J. L., DUBOISSET, M., LESBRE, P. and BERNASCONI, P., Diphenylhydantoin injectable in cardiology, *Arch. Mal. Coeur.*, 67: 87-96, 1974.   *27*

1435. RAINES, A. and STANDAERT, F. G., Effects of anticonvulsant drugs on nerve terminals, *Epilepsia*, 10: 211-227, 1969.

1436. RAINES, A., LEVITT, B., STANDAERT, F. G., and SOHN, Y. J., The influence of sympathetic nervous activity on the antiarrhythmic efficacy of diphenylhydantoin, *Europ. J. Pharmacol.*, 11: 293-297, 1970.

1437. RAINES, A., SOHN, Y. J., and LEVITT, B., Spinal excitatory and depressant effects of sodium diphenylthiohydantoinate, *J. Pharmacol. Exp. Ther.*, 177: 350-359, 1971.

1438. RAINES, A., Effects of diphenylhydantoin on post-tetanic alterations in the terminals of dorsal root fibers and motor nerves, *Georgetown University Doctoral Thesis*, June, 1965.

1439. RALSTON, A. J., SNAITH, R. P., and HINLEY, J. B., Effects of folic acid on fit-frequency and behaviour in epileptics on anticonvulsants, *Lancet*, 1: 867-868, 1970.

1440. RAMDOHR, VON B., SCHUREN, K. P., DENNERT, J., MACHA, H.-N. and SCHRODER, R., Influence of diphenylhydantoin on hemodynamics in recent myocardial infarct., *Verhandlungen der Deutschen Gesellschaft fur Kreislaufforschung*, 35: 444-50, 1969.

1441. RANE, A., GARLE, M., BORGA, O., SJOQVIST, F., Plasma disappearance of transplacentally transferred diphenylhydantoin in the newborn studied with mass fragmentography, *Clin. Pharmacol. Ther.* 15: 39-45, 1974.

1442. RANE, A., LUNDE, P. K. M., JALLING, B., et al, Plasma protein binding of diphenylhydantoin in normal and hyperbilirubinemic infants, *Epilepsy Abstracts*, 4: 223, 1971.

1443. RANE, A., Urinary excretion of diphenylhydantoin metabolites in newborn infants, *J. Pediat.*, 85: 543-545, 1974.

1444. RASKIN, N. H., LEVINSON, S. A., PICKETT, J. B., HOFFMAN, P. M., and FIELDS, H. L., Postsympathectomy   *37* neuralgia, *Amer. J. Surg.*, 128: 75-78, 1974.

1445. RASKOVIC, J., Phenomenological aspects of the psychotic epileptic state in terms of therapeutic argument, *Neuropsihialrya*, 20: 161-166, 1972.

1446. RAY, A. K. and RAO, D. B., Calcium metabolism in elderly epileptic patients during anticonvulsant therapy, *Epilepsy Abstracts*, 7: 210, 1974.

1447. RAZ, S., ZEIGLER, M., and CAINE, M., The effect of diphenylhydantoin on the urethra, *Invest. Urol.*, 10: 293-294, 1973.

1448. REIDENBERG, M. M., ODAR-CEDERLOF, I., VON BAHR, C., BORGA, O., and SJOQVIST, F., Protein binding of diphenylhydantoin and desmethylimipramine in plasma from patients with poor renal function, *New Eng., J. Med.*, 285: 264-267, 1971.

1449. REIMANN, H. A., Abdominal epilepsy and migraine, *JAMA*, 224: 128, 1973.

1450. REIMANN, R., LEMMEL, W., and THEISEN, K., Efficacy and risks of diphenylhydantoin in cardiac arrhyth-   *24* mias, *Munchen Med. Wschr.*, 113: 893-899, 1971.

1451. REIZENSTEIN, P. and LUND, L., Effect of anticonvulsive drugs on folate absorption and the cerebrospinal folate pump, *Epilepsy Abstracts*, 7: 86, 1974.

1452. REMMER, H., Induction of drug metabolizing enzyme system in the liver, *Eur. J. Clin. Pharmacol.*, 5: 116-136, 1972.

1453. RESNEKOV, L., Drug therapy before and after the electroversion of cardiac dysrhythmias, *Progr. Cardiovasc. Dis.*, 16: 531-538, 1974.

1454. RETTURA, G., STAMFORD, W. and SEIFTER, E., Reversal of cardiac calcification by diphenylhydantoin,   *33* *Paper presented at N.E. Regional Meeting of the American Chemical Society*, Oct., 1973.

1455. REYNOLDS, E. H., Anticonvulsant drugs, folic acid metabolism and schizophrenia-like psychoses in epilepsy, *Psychische Storungen bei Epilepsie*, H. Penin, Ed., F. K. Schattauer Verlag, Stuttgart-New York, 1973.

1456. REYNOLDS, E. H., Anticonvulsant drugs, folic acid metabolism, fit frequency and psychiatric illness, *Psychiat. Neurol. Neurochir.*, 74: 167-174, 1971.

1457. REYNOLDS, E. H., Anticonvulsants, folic acid and epilepsy, *Lancet*, 1376-1378, June, 1973.

1458. REYNOLDS, E. H., CHANARIN, I., MILNER, G. and MATTHEWS, D. M., Anticonvulsant therapy, folic acid and vitamin B^{12} metabolism and mental symptoms, *Epilepsia*, 7: 261-270, 1966.

1459. REYNOLDS, E. H., MATTSON, R., and GALLAGHER, B., Relationships between serum and cerebrospinal fluid anticonvulsant drug and folic acid concentrations in epileptic patients, *Neurology*, 22: 841-844, 1972.

1460. REYNOLDS, E. H., STREIFF, R. R., WILDER, B. J., and HAMMER, R. H., Diphenylhydantoin hematologic aspects of toxicity, *Antiepilepic Drugs*, 247-266, Woodbury, D. M., Penry, J. K., and Schmidt, R. P., Eds., Raven Press, New York, 1972. (*cf.* Bottomley, et al., *J. Mich. Dent. Ass.*, 53: 256, 1971 and Kolodzieczak and Prazanowski, *Epilepsy Abstracts*, 5: 149, 1972.)

1461. REYNOLDS, J. W. and MIRKIN, B. L., Urinary corticosteroid and diphenylhydantoin metabolite patterns in neonates exposed to anticonvulsant drugs in utero, *JAMA*, 227: 577, 1974.

1462. RHEE, R. S., MARGOLIN, M., and PELLOCK, J., Palatal myoclonus and diphenylhydantoin therapy, *New*   *47* *Eng. J. Med.*, 290: 1088-1089, 1974.

1463. RICHENS, A. and HOUGHTON, G. W., Phenytoin intoxication caused by sulthiame, *Lancet*, 1442-1443, 1973.

1464. RICHENS, A. and ROWE, D. J. F., Disturbance of calcium metabolism by anticonvulsant drugs, *Brit. Med. J.*, 4: 73-76, 1970.

1465. RICHENS, A. and ROWE, D. J. F., Anticonvulsant hypocalcaemia, *Epilepsy Abstracts*, 5: 224, 1972.

REFERENCES

1466. RIDDELL, D. and LEONARD, B. E., Some properties of a coma producing material obtained from mammalian brain, *Neuropharmacology*, 9: 283-299, 1970.   *86*

1467. RIEHL, J. L. and McINTYRE, H. B., Acute effects of Dilantin on the EEG of epileptic patients: a quantitative study, *Electroenceph. Clin. Neurophysiol.*, 28: 94, 1970.   *60*

1468. RIFKIND, A. B., GILLETTE, P. N., SONG, C. S., and KAPPAS, A., Drug stimulation of ∂-Aminolevulinic acid synthetase and cytochrome P-450 *in vivo* in chick embryo liver, *J. Pharmacol. Exp. Ther.* 185: 214-225, 1973.

1469. RIKER, W. F., The pharmacology of the neostigmine-like facilitatory drug effect at the mammalian neuromuscular junction, *Jap. J. Pharmacol.*, 22: 1, 1972.   *61*

1470. RISH, B. L. and CAVENESS, W. F., Relation of prophylactic medication to the occurrence of early seizures following craniocerebral trauma, *J. Neurosurg.*, 38: 155-158, 1973.

1471. RIZZO, M., MORSELLI, P. L., and GARATTINI, S., Further observations on the interactions between phenobarbital and diphenylhydantoin during chronic treatment in the rat, *Biochem. Pharmacol.*, 21: 449-454, 1972.   *92*

1472. ROBBINS, M. M., Aplastic anemia secondary to anticonvulsants, *Amer. J. Dis. Child.*, 104: 64-74, 1962.

1473. ROBERTS, E., An hypothesis suggesting that there is a defect in the GABA system in schizophrenia, *Neurosciences Research Program Bulletin*, 10: 468-482, 1972.

1474. ROBERTS, J., The effect of diphenylhydantoin on the response to accelerator nerve stimulation, *Proc. Soc. Exp. Biol. Med.*, 134: 274-280, 1970.

1475. ROBINEAUX, R., LORANS, G., and BEAURE D'AUGERES, C., Action of diphenylhydantoin on the growth and respiration of cell in culture, *Rev. Europ. Etudes Clin. Biol.*, 15: 1066-1071, 1970.

1476. ROCKLIFF, B. W. and DAVIS, E. H., Controlled sequential trials of carbamazepine in trigeminal neuralgia, *Arch. Neurol.*, 15: 129-136, 1966.

1477. RODMAN, N. F., McDEVITT, N. B., and ALMOND, J. R., Platelet function inhibition by diphenylhydantoin, *Fed. Proc.*, 30: Abstract 513, 1971.

1478. ROMAN, I. C. and CARATZALI, A., Effects of anticonvulsant drugs on chromosomes, *Brit. Med. J.*, 234, 1971.

1479. ROMERO, E., MARANON, A. and BOBILLO, E. R., Antithyroid action of hydantoin derivatives, *Rev. Iber. Endocr.*, 101: 363-375, 1970.   *49*

1480. ROSE, L. I., WILLIAMS, G. H., JAGGER, P. I., LAULER, D. P., and THORN, G. W., The paradoxical dexamethasone response phenomenon, *Metabolism*, 18: 369-375, 1969.   *29*

1481. ROSENTHAL, J. E. and COHEN, L. S., Therapeutic predicament—the unresponsive PVC, *Geriatrics*, 28: 88-92, 1973.

1482. ROSS, G. S., A technique to study pain in monkeys; effect of drugs and anatomic lesions, *Henry Ford Hosp. Symposium on Pain*, Chap. 8, 100-101, Knighton, R. S. and Dumke, P. R., Eds., Little, Brown and Co., Boston, 1966.

1483. ROSS, G. S., Effect of diphenylhydantoin on experimental pain in the monkey, *Neurology*, 15: 275, 1965.   *91*

1484. ROSS, L. M., Diphenylhydantoin (DPH) induced cleft palate, *Teratology*, 7: A-26, June, 1973.

1485. ROVIN, S., SABES, W. R., EVERSOLE, L. R., and GORDON, H. A., Dilantin as a caries retarder, *J. Dent. Res.*, 52: 267, 1973.   *90*

1486. RUBINS, S., LOZANO, J., CARRASCO, H., LANG, T. W., and CORDAY, E., Tachyarrhythmias: Differential diagnosis and therapy after acute myocardial infarction, *Geriatrics*, 27: 123-133, 1972.

1487. RUDNER, E. J., Diphenylhydantoin therapy, *Arch. Derm.*, 102: 561, 1970.

1488. RUMACK, B. H., WOLFE, R. R. and GILFRICH, H., Phenytoin (diphenylhydantoin) treatment of massive digoxin overdose, *Brit. Heart J.*, 36: 405-408, 1974.   *24*

1489. RUNDLE, A. T. and SUDELL, B., Leucine aminopeptidase isoenzyme changes after treatment with anticonvulsant drugs, *Clin. Chim. Acta*, 44: 377-384, 1973.

1490. RUSHTON, J. G., Medical treatment of trigeminal neuralgia, *Med. Clin. N. Amer.*, 52: 797-800, 1968.

1491. RUSKIN, H. M., Therapeutic Dilantin levels, *New Eng., J. Med.*, 284: 792, 1971.

1492. RUTKOWSKI, M. M., COHEN, S. N., and DOYLE, E. F., Drug therapy of heart disease in pediatric patients. II. The treatment of congestive heart failure in infants and children with digitalis preparations, _Amer. Heart J._, 86: 270-275, 1973.

1493. RUTKOWSKI, M. M., DOYLE, E. F., and COHEN, S. N., Drug therapy of heart disease in pediatric patients III. The therapeutic challenge of supraventricular tachyarrhythmias in infants and children, _Amer. Heart J._, 86: 562-568, 1973.

1494. RUTLEDGE, R., SOHN, Y. J., and SARDINAS, A., Interaction of diphenylhydantoin and succinylcholine at the neuromuscular junction, _Pharmacologist_, 13: 265, 1971.   _70_

1495. SAAD, S. F., EL MASRY, A. M., and SCOTT, P. M., Influence of certain anticonvulsants on the concentration of 8-aminobutyric acid in the cerebral hemispheres of mice, _Communications in Behav. Biol._, 9: February, 1972.   _79_

1496. SABIH, K. and SABIH, K., Combined GLC and high-resolution mass spectroscopic analysis of diphenylhydantoin, _J. Pharm. Sci._, 60: 1216-1220, 1971.

1497. SAMPLINER, R., Diphenylhydantoin control of alcohol withdrawal seizures, _JAMA_, 230: 1430-1432, 1974.

1498. SAMPSON, D., HARASYMIV, I., and HENSLEY, W. J., Gas chromatographic assay of underivatized 5,5-diphenylhydantoin (Dilantin) in plasma extracts, _Clin. Chem._, 17: 382-385, 1971.

1499. SANO, T., SUZUKI, F., SATO, S., and IIDA, Y., Mode of action of new anti-arrhythmic agents, _Jap. Heart J._, 9: 161-168, 1968.

1500. SATALINE, L., Cardiac standstill simulating epileptic seizures, _JAMA_, 225: 747, 1973.

1501. SATOYOSHI, E. and YAMADA, K., Recurrent muscle spasms of central origin. A report of two cases, _Arch. Neurol._, 16: 254-264, 1967.   _45_

1502. SATOYOSHI, E., Recurrent muscle spasms of central origin, _Trans. Amer. Neurol. Assoc._, 92: 153-157, 1967.

1503. SAUNDERS, B. A. and JENKINS, L. C., Cardiac arrhythmias of central nervous system origin: possible mechanism and suppression, _Canad. Anaesth. Soc. J._, 20: 617-628, 1973.

1504. SAVINI, E. C., POITEVIN, R., and POITEVIN, J., New treatment of periodontolysis, _Rev. Franc Odontostomat._, 19: 55-61, 1972.   _51_

1505. SCHADE, G. H. and GOFMAN, H., Abdominal epilepsy in childhood, _Pediatrics_, 25: 151-154, 1960.

1506. SCHERLAG, B. J. and HELFANT, R. H., Effect of diphenylhydantoin on acetyl strophanthidin, _Amer. Heart J._, 81(4): 577-579, 1971.

1507. SCHERLAG, B. J., HELFANT, R. H., RICCIUTTI, M. A., DAMATO, A. N., Dissociation of the effects of digitalis on myocardial potassium flux and contractility, _Am. J. Physiology_, 215: 1288-1291, 1968.   _34_

1508. SCHICK, D. and SCHEUER, J., Current concepts of therapy with digitalis glycosides, Part II., _Amer. Heart J._, 87: 391-396, 1974.   _86_

1509. SCHIMMEL, R. J. and GRAHAM, D., Inhibition by diphenylhydantoin of the diabetogenic action of streptozotocin, _Horm. Metab. Res._, 6: 475-477, 1974.   _84_

1510. SCHOOR, W. P., Effect of anticonvulsant drugs on insecticide residues, _Lancet_, 520-521, 1970.   _85_

1511. SCHREIBER, M. M. and McGREGOR, J. G., Pseudolymphoma syndrome, _Arch. Derm._, 97: 297-300, 1968.

1512. SCHULTEN, H. K., ETZRODT, H., DU MESNIL DE ROCHEMONT, W., CHRISKE, H. W., GROSSER, K. D., and STEINBRUCK, G., Clinical and electrophysiological observations in DPH therapy of arrhythmia, _Verh. Deutsch Ges. Inn. Med._, 77: 952-956, 1971.

1513. SCHUSSLER, G. C., Diazepam competes for thyroxine binding sites, _Chem. Abstracts_, 75: 74395C, 1971.

1514. SCHUSSLER, G. C., Similarity of diazepam to diphenylhydantoin, _JAMA_, 218: 1832, 1971.

1515. SCHWENDER, C. F., Antiarrhythmic agents, _Annual Reports in Medicinal Chemistry, 1970_, 80-87, Cain, C. K., Ed., Academic Press, New York, 1971.   _86_

1516. SCIENTIFIC REVIEW SUBPANEL ON ANTIARRHYTHMIA AGENTS, Quinidine-reserpine, Evaluations of Drug Interactions, _American Pharmaceutical Association_, Washington, D. C., 130-131, 1973.

1517. SCIENTIFIC REVIEW SUBPANEL ON ANTICONVULSANTS, Diphenylhydantoin—Isoniazid, Evaluations of Drug Interactions, _American Pharmaceutical Association_, Washington, D. C., 51-52, 1973.

REFERENCES

1518. Scientific Review Subpanel on Anticonvulsants, Diphenylhydantoin—phenobarbital, Evaluations of Drug Interactions, *American Pharmaceutical Association*, Washington, D. C., 54-56, 1973.

1519. Scientific Review Subpanel on Antidiabetic Agents, Insulin-diphenylhydantoin, *Evaluations of Drug Interaction*, American Pharmaceutical Association, Washington, D.C., 90-91, 1973.

1520. Scientific Review Subpanel on Anticonvulsants, Diphenylhydantoin-Methylphenidate, Evaluations of Drug Interactions, *American Pharmaceutical Association*, Washington, D.C., 53-54, 1973.

1521. Scientific Review Subpanel on Steroids, Dexamethasone-diphenylhydantoin, Evaluations of Drug Interactions, *American Pharmaceutical Association*, Washington, D. C., 32-34, 1973.

1522. Scientific Review Subpanel on Anticonvulsants, Anticonvulsant therapy, Evaluations of Drug Interactions, *American Pharmaceutical Association*, Washington, D.C., 252-256, 1973.

1523. Scott, M., Peale, A. R., and Croissant, P. D., Intracranial midline anterior fossae ossifying fibroma invading orbits, paranasal sinuses, and right maxillary antrum, *J. Neurosurg.*, 34: 827-831, 1971.

1524. Seeman, P., Chau-Wong, M., and Moyyen, S., The membrane binding of morphine, diphenylhydantoin, and tetrahydrocannabinol, *Canad. J. Physiol. Pharmacol.*, 50: 1193-1200, 1972.

1525. Selye, H. and Szabo, S., Protection by various steroids against gold nephropathy, *J. Europ. Toxicol.*, 6: 512-516, 1972.   *86*

1526. Selye, H. and Tuchweber, B., Effect of various steroids upon the toxicity of bile acids, *Int. Symp. Hepatotoxicity*, 63, 1973.

1527. Selye, H., Szabo, S., and Kourounakis, P., Effect of various steroids and nonsteroidal microsomal enzyme inducers upon propoxyphene intoxication, *Neuroendocrinology*, 9: 316-319, 1972.   *87*

1528. Selye, H., Szabo, S., and Kourounakis, P., Protection against phenylisothicyanate by various steroids, phenobarbitone and diphenylhydantoin, *J. Pharm. Pharmacol.*, 24: 333-334, 1972.   *87*

1529. Selye, H., Szabo, S., and Kourounakis, P., Protection by catatoxic steroids, phenobarbital and diphenylhydantoin against methaqualone intoxication, *Steroids Lipids Res.*, 3: 156-159, 1972.   *86*

1530. Selye, H., Szabo, S., and Mecs, I., Protection by catatoxic steroids against the paralysis caused by combined treatment with thyroxine and methylphenidate, *Neuropharmacology*, 11: 693-696, 1972.   *86*

1531. Selye, H., Hormones and resistance, *J. Pharm. Sci.*, 60: 1-28, 1971.

1532. Selye, H., Prevention by catatoxic steroids of lithocholic acid-induced biliary concrements in the rat, *Proc. Soc. Exp. Biol. Med.*, 141: 555-558, 1972.

1533. Selye, H., Protection by glucocorticoids against allopurinol nephropathy, *Acta Endocr.*, 69: 347-354, 1972.

1534. Serrano, E. E., Roye, D. B., Hammer, R. H., and Wilder, B. J., Plasma diphenylhydantoin values after oral and intramuscular administration of diphenylhydantoin, *Neurology*, 23: 311-317, 1973.

1535. Shah, J. R., Vora, G., Karkhanis, A. V., and Talwalkar, C. V., The effect of diphenylhydantoin on ventilation tests in airway obstruction, *Indian J. Chest. Dis.*, 12: 10-14, 1970.   *48*

1536. Shalsha, K. G., The function of newer antiarrhythmic drugs under special consideration of beta blocking adrenergic agents, *Proc. Virchow Med. Soc. N. Y.*, 27: 201-211, 1969.

1537. Shemano, I., Orzechowski, R., Goldstein, S., and Beiler, J. M., Effects of 3,5-diethylhydantoin on resistance to asphyxia in rats, *Toxic. Appl. Pharmacol.* 25: 250-258, 1973.

1538. Sher, S. P., Drug enzyme induction and drug interactions: literature tabulation, *Toxic. Appl. Pharmacol.*, 18: 780-834, 1971.

1539. Sherwin, A. L., Eisen, A. A. and Sokolowski, C. D., Anticonvulsant drugs in human epileptogenic brain, *Presented at the annual meeting of the American Neurological Association and the Canadian Congress of Neurological Sciences*, Montreal, 1973.   *92*

1540. Sherwin, I., Suppressant effects of diphenylhydantoin on the cortical epileptogenic focus, *Neurology*, 23: 274-281, 1973.

1541. Shibasaki, H. and Kuroiwa, Y., Painful tonic seizure in multiple sclerosis, *Arch. Neurol.*, 30: 47-51, 1974.

1542. Shinohara, Y., Ventricular fibrillation threshold (VFRT) in experimental coronary occlusion: comparative studies on the effect of G-I-K solution and some new antiarrhythmic agents, *Jap. Circ. J.*, 32: 1269-1281, 1968.

1543. SHOEMAN, D. W., BENJAMIN, D. M., and AZARNOFF, D. L., The alteration of plasma proteins in uremia as reflected in the ability to bind diphenylhydantoin, *Ann. N. Y. Acad. Sci.*, 226: 127-130, 1973.

1544. SHOEMAN, D. W., KAUFFMAN, R. E., AZARNOFF, D. L., and BOULOS, B. M., Placental transfer of diphenyl-hydantoin as determined at constant drug concentrations in the maternal blood, *Pharmacologist*, 13: 195, 1971.

1545. SHOEMAN, D. W., KAUFFMAN, R. E., AZARNOFF, D. L., and BOULOS, B. M., Placental transfer of diphenyl-hydantoin in the goat, *Biochem. Pharmacol.*, 21: 1237-1244, 1972.

1546. SHOLITON, L. J., WERK, E. E. and MacGEE, J., The effect of diphenylhydantoin *in vitro* on the formation of the polar metabolites of testosterone by rat liver, *Acta Endocr.*, 62: 360-366, 1969.

1547. SIEGEL, G. H. and GOODWIN, B. B., Sodium-potassium-activated adenosine triphosphatase of brain microsomes: modification of sodium inhibition by diphenylhydantoins, *J. Clin. Invest.*, 51: 1161-1169, 1972.

1548. SIEGEL, G. J. and GOODWIN, B. B., Effects of 5,5-diphenylhydantoin (DPH) and 5-p-hydroxyphenyl-5-phenylhydantoin (HPPH) on brain Na-K-ATPase, *Neurology*, 21: 417, 1971.

1549. SIGWALD, J., RAVERDY, P., FARDEAU, M., GREMY, F., MACE DE LEPINAY, A., BOUTTIER, D., and DANIC, Mme., Pseudo-myotonia, *Rev. Neurol.*, 115: 1003-1014, 1966.

1550. SIMON, G. E., JATLOW, P. I., SELIGSON, H. T., and SELIGSON, D., Measurement of 5,5-diphenylhydantoin in blood using thin layer chromatography, *Elilepsy* Abstracts, 4: 136, 1971.

1551. SIMOPOULOS, A. M. PINTO, A., UHLENHUTH, E. H., McGEE, J. J., and DeROSA, E. R., Diphenylhydantoin (DPH) effectiveness in the treatment of chronic schizophrenics, *Arch. Gen. Psychiat.*, 30: 106-112, 1974.

1552. SIMPSON, J. F., Use of diphenylhydantoin, *Ann. Intern. Med.*, 78: 305-306, 1973.

1553. SINGH, B. N. and HAUSWIRTH, O., Comparative mechanisms of action of antiarrhythmic drugs, *Amer. Heart J.*, 87: 367-382, 1974.

1554. SINGH, B. N. and VAUGHAN WILLIAMS, E. M., Effect of altering potassium concentration on the action of lidocaine and diphenylhydantoin on rabbit atrial and ventricular muscle, *Circ. Res.*, 29: 286-295, 1971.

1555. SINGH, B. N., Explanation for the discrepancy in reported cardiac electrophysiological actions of diphenylhydantoin and lignocaine, *Brit. J. Pharmacol.*, 41: 385-386, 1971.

1556. SINGH, H. P., HEBERT, M. A., and GUALT, M. H., Effect of some drugs on clinical laboratory values as determined by technicon SMA 12/60, *Clin. Chem.*, 18: 137-144, 1972.

1557. SINGH, N., SINHA, J. N., RASTOGI, S. K., DUA, P. R., and KOHLI, R. P., An experimental investigation on the antiarrhythmic activity of antiepileptic agents, *Jap. J. Pharmacol.* 21: 755-761, 1971.   *31*

1558. SISCA, T. S., An unusual dual hypersensitivity reaction induced by diphenylhydantoin, *Amer. J. Hosp. Pharm.*, 30: 446-449, 1973.

1559. SKROTSKY, Y. A., Complications due to antiepileptic therapy in children and adolescents, *Epilepsy Abstracts*, 7: 138-139, 1974.

1560. SLOSBERG, P. S., Medical therapy for the cerebrovascular insufficiencies: eight years' experience, *Mt. Sinai Med. J.*, 37: 692-698, 1970.   *29*

1561. SMITH, J. S., BRIERLEY, H. and BRANDON, S., Akinetic mutism with recovery after repeated carbon monoxide poisoning, *Psychol. Med.*, 1: 172-177, 1971.

1562. SMITH, T. W. and HABER, E., Digitalis, *New Eng. J. Med.*, 289: 1125-1129, 1973.   *23*

1563. SMITH, T. W., Digitalis glycosides, *New Eng. J. Med.*, 288: 942-946, 1973.   *86*

1564. SMITH, W. L. and LOWREY, J. B., The effects of diphenylhydantoin on cognitive functions in man, *Drugs, Development, and Cerebral Function*, Smith, W. L., Ed., Charles C. Thomas, 344-351, 1972.   *17*

1565. SMITH, W. L. and LOWREY, J. B., The effects of diphenylhydantoin on concentration in the elderly, *J. Amer. Geriat. Soc.* (In press), 1975.   *18*

1566. SNIDER, R. S. and DEL CERRO, M., Diphenylhydantoin, proliferating membranes in cerebellum resulting from intoxication, *Antiepileptic Drugs*, 237-245, WOODBURY, D. M., PENRY, J. K., and SCHMIDT, R. P. Eds., Raven Press, New York, 1972.

1567. SOHN, R. S. and FERRENDELLI, J. A., Inhibition of Ca^{++}, uptake in rat brain synaptosomes by diphenylhydantoin, *Neurology*, 23: 444, 1973.   *77*

REFERENCES

1568. SOLOMON, G. E., HILGARTNER, M. W., and KUTT, H., Coagulation defects caused by diphenylhydantoin, *Neurology,* 22: 1165-1171, 1972.

1569. SOLOMON, P. and KLEEMAN, S. T., Medical aspects of violence, *Calif. Med.,* 114: 19-24, 1971. *16*

1570. SOLOW, E. B. and GREEN, J. B., The simultaneous determination of multiple anticonvulsant drug levels by gas-liquid chromatography, *Neurology,* 22: 540-550, 1972.

1571. SOLOW, E. B., METAXAS, J. M. and SUMMERS, T. R., Antiepileptic drugs. A current assessment of simultaneous determination of multiple drug therapy by gas liquid chromatography-on column methylation, *J. Chromatographic Sci.,* 12: 256-260, 1974.

1572. SORRELL, T. C., FORBES, I. J., BURNESS, F. R., and RISCHBIETH, R. H. C., Depression of immunological function in patients treated with phenytoin sodium (sodium diphenylhydantoin), *Lancet,* 1233-1235, 1971.

1573. SOTANIEMI, E. A., ARVELA, P., HAKKARAINEN, H. K., and HUHTI, E., The clinical significance of microsomal enzyme induction in the therapy of epileptic patients, *Ann. Clin. Res.,* 2: 223-227, 1970.

1574. SOTANIEMI, E. A., HAKKARAINEN, H. K., PURANEN, J. A., and LAHTI, R. O., Radiologic bone changes and hypocalcemia with anticonvulsant therapy in epilepsy, *Ann. Intern. Med.,* 77(3): 389-394, 1972.

1575. SOUTH, J., Teratogenic effect of anticonvulsants, *Lancet,* 2: 1154, 1972.

1576. SPECTOR, R. G., Effects of formyl tetrahydrofolic acid and noradrenaline on the oxygen consumption of   *67*
rat brain synaptosome-mitrochondrial preparations, *Brit. J. Pharmacol.,* 44: 279-285, 1972.

1577. SPECTOR, R. G., Influence of folic acid on excitable tissues, *Nature New Biol.,* 240: 247-249, 1972.

1578. SPECTOR, R. G., The influence of anticonvulsant drugs on formyl tetrahydrofolic acid stimulation of rat brain respiration *in vitro, Epilepsy Abstracts,* 6: 110, 1973.

1579. SPEIDEL, B. D. and MEADOW, S. R., Maternal epilepsy and abnormalities of the fetus and newborn, *Lancet,* 839-843, October, 1972.

1580. SPERELAKIS, N. and HENN, F. A., Effect of diphenylhydantoin on membrane potentials and Na-K-ATPase   *31*
of cultured chick heart cells, *Amer. J. Physiol.,* 218: 1224-1227, 1970.

1581. SPINA, A., Pyridinolcarbamate in the therapy of hemicrania syndromes, *Acta Neurol.,* 27: 610-617, 1972.

1582. SPRAY, G. H. and BURNS, D. G., Folate deficiency and anticonvulsant drugs, *Brit. Med. J.,* 2: 167-168, April, 1972.

1583. STAMBAUGH, J. E. and TUCKER, D., Effect of diphenylhydantoin on glucose tolerance in patients with   *10*
hypoglycemia, *Diabetes,* 23: 679-683, 1974.

1584. STAMP, T. C. B., Effects of long-term anticonvulsant therapy on calcium and vitamin D metabolism, *Proc. Roy. Soc. Med.,* 67: 64-68, 1974.

1585. STAMP, T. C. B., ROUND, J. M., ROWE, D. J. F., and HADDAD, J. G., Plasma levels and therapeutic effect of 25-hydroxycholecalciferol in epileptic patients taking anticonvulsant drugs, *Brit. Med. J.,* 4: 9-12, 1972.

1586. STAPLES, R. E., Teratology, *Antiepileptic Drugs,* 55-62, WOODBURY, D. M., PENRY, J. K., and SCHMIDT, R. P. Eds., Raven Press, New York, 1972. (*cf.* Kuenssberg and Knox, *Lancet,* 198, 1973. Millar and Nevin, *Lancet,* 328, 1973 and Stenchever and Jarvis, *Amer. J. Obstet. Gynec.,* 109: 961, 1971.)

1587. STARREVELD-ZIMMERMAN, A. A. E., VAN DER KOLK, W. J., MEINARDI, H., and ELSHOVE, J., Are anticonvulsants teratogenic?, *Lancet,* 48-49, July, 1973.

1588. STAUNTON, C., STEIN, A. A., and MOSS, G., The cerebral etiology of the respiratory distress syndrome (RDS): universal response, with prevention by unilateral pulmonary denervation, *Surg. Forum,* 24: 1973.

1589. STAVCHANSKY, S. A., LUBAWY, W. C. and KOSTENBAUDER, H. B., Increase of hexobarbital sleeping time and inhibition of drug metabolism by the major metabolite of DPH, *Life Sci.,* 14: 1535-1539, 1974.

1590. STAZI, C. and MARASA, G., Arrhythmias due to digitalis and their treatment, *Ann. Med. Nav.* (Roma), 77:   *23*
51-80, 1972.

1591. STEIN, A. A. and MOSS, G., Cerebral etiology of the respiratory distress syndrome: diphenylhydantoin   *68*
(DPH) prophylaxis, *Surg. Forum,* 24: 433-435, 1973.

1592. STEPHENS, J. H. and SHAFFER, J. W., A controlled replication of the effectiveness of diphenylhydantoin in   *14*
reducing irritability and anxiety in selected neurotic outpatients, *J. Clin. Pharmacol.,* 13: 351-356, 1973.

1593. STEPHENS, J. H., SHAFFER, J. W., and BROWN, C. C., A controlled comparison of the effects of diphenylhy- *88*
dantoin and placebo on mood and psychomotor functioning in normal volunteers, *J. Clin. Pharma-col.*, 14: 543-551, 1974.

1594. STERN, L. Z., GRUENER, R., and AMUNDSEN, P., Diphenylhydantoin for steroid-induced muscle weakness, *44*
JAMA, 223: 1287-1288, 1973.

1595. STEVENS, H., Nine neuropathies, *Med. Ann.*, 37: 89-97, 1968.

1596. STEVENS, M. W. and HARBISON, R. D., Placental transfer of diphenylhydantoin: effects of species, gestational age, and route of administration, *Teratology*, 9: 317-326, 1974.

1597. STEVENSON, M. M. and GILBERT, E. F., Anticonvulsants and hemorrhagic diseases of the newborn infant, *J. Pediat.*, 516, 1970.

1598. STONE, N., KLEIN, M. D., and LOWN, B., Diphenylhydantoin in the prevention of recurring ventricular *25*
tachycardia, *Circulation*, 43: 420-427, 1971.

1599. STOWELL, A., Physiologic mechanisms and treatment of histaminic or petrosal neuralgia, *Headache*, 9: 187-194, 1970.

1600. STRAUSS, H., RAHM, W. E., and BARRERA, S. E., Studies on a group of children with psychiatric disorders. I. Electroencephalographic studies, *Psychosom. Med.*, 2: 34-42, 1940.

1601. STRITTMATTER, W. J. and SOMJEN, G. G., Depression of sustained evoked potentials and glial depolarization in the spinal cord by barbiturates and by diphenylhydantoin, *Brain Res.*, 55: 333-342, 1973.

1602. SU, P. C. and FELDMAN, D. S., Motor nerve terminal and muscle membrane stabilization by diphenylhy- *61*
dantoin administration, *Arch. Neurol.*, 28: 376-379, 1973.

1603. SWAIMAN, K. F. and STRIGHT, P. L., The effects of anticonvulsants on *in vitro* protein synthesis in immature brain, *Brain Res.*, 58: 515-518, 1973.

1604. SWANN, W. P., Effects of dilantin on the repair of gingival wounds, *Indiana University School of Dentistry, Thesis*, 1966.

1605. SWEET, W. H. and WEPSIC, J. G., Relation of fiber size in trigeminal posterior root to conduction of impulses for pain and touch; production of analgesia without anesthesia in the effective treatment of trigeminal neuralgia, *Trans. Amer. Neurol. Assoc.*, 95: 134-139, 1970.

1606. TABACHNICK, M., HAO, Y. L., and KORCEK, L., Effect of oleate, diphenylhydantoin and heparin on the binding of 125 I-thyroxine to purified thyroxine-binding globulin, *J. Clin. Endocr.*, 36: 392-394, 1973.

1607. TAITZ, L. S., Mental retardation elevated alkaline phosphatase, convulsive disorder and thickening of calvarium, *Epilepsy Abstracts*, 6: 228, 1973. (*cf.* Kattan, *Amer. J. Roentgen.*, 110: 102, 1970.)

1608. TAPPAZ, M. and PACHECO, H., Effects of convulsant and anticonvulsant drugs on uptake of 14,-C GABA *93*
by rat brain slices, *J. Pharmacol.* (Paris), 4: 295-306, 1973.

1609. TASHIMA, C. K. and DE LOS SANTOS, R., Lymphoma and anticonvulsive therapy, *JAMA*, 228: 286-287, 1974.

1610. TASSINARI, C. A. and FINE, R. D., Paroxysmal choreoathetosis, *Proc. Aust. Assoc. Neurol.*, 6: 71-75, 1969. *43*

1611. TAYLOR, C. R., Double-blind crossover study of diphenylhydantoin in angina pectoris, *Chest*, 66: 422- *27*
427, 1974.

1612. TAYLOR, J. D., KRAHN, P. M. and HIGGINS, T. N., Serum copper levels and diphenylhydantoin, *Amer. J. Clin. Path.*, 61: 577-578, 1974.

1613. TENSER, R. B. and CORBETT, J. J., Myokymia and facial contraction in brain stem glioma, *Arch. Neurol.*, *47*
30: 425-427, 1974.

1614. THOMPSON, C. E., Diphenylhydantoin for myotonia congenita, *New Eng. J. Med.*, 286: 893, 1972. *43*

1615. THURKOW, I., WESSELING, H., and MEIJER, D. K. F., Estimation of phenytoin in body fluids in the presence of sulphonyl urea compounds, *Clin. Chim. Acta*, 37: 509-513, 1972.

1616. THURLOW, H. J. and GIRVIN, J. P., Use of anti-epileptic medication in treating "flashbacks" from *19*
hallucinogenic drugs, *Canad. Med. Assoc. J.*, 105: 947-948, 1971.

1617. TIGELAAR, R. E., RAPPORT, R. L., INMAN, J. K., and KUPFERBERG, H. J., A radioimmunoassay for diphenylhydantoin, *Epilepsy Abstracts*, 6: 113, 1973.

REFERENCES

1618. TISMAN, G., HERBERT, V., GO, L. T., and BRENNER, L., *In vitro* demonstration of immunosuppression without bone marrow suppression by alcohol and bleomycin, *Clin. Res.*, 19: 730, 1971.

1619. TOBIN, T., DIRDJOSUDJONO, S., and BASKIN, S. I., Pharmacokinetics and distribution of diphenylhydantoin in kittens, *Amer. J. Vet. Res.*, 34: 951-954, 1973.

1620. TOLMAN, K. G., JUBIZ, W., DeLUCA, H. F. and FRESTON, J. W., Rickets associated with anticonvulsant medications, *Clin. Res.*, 20: 414, 1972.

1621. TOMAN, J. E. P. and SABELLI, H. C., Comparative neuronal mechanisms, *Epilepsia*, 10: 179-192, 1969.

1622. TORRETTI, J., HENDLER, E., WEINSTEIN, E., LONGNECKER, R. E., and EPSTEIN, F. H., Functional significance of Na-K-ATPase in the kidney: effects of ouabain inhibition, *Amer. J. Physiol.*, 222: 1398-1405. 1972.   *86*

1623. TOVI, D., The use of antifibrinolytic drugs to prevent early recurrent aneurysmal subarachnoid haemorrhage, *Acta Neurol. Scand.*, 49: 163-175, 1973.

1624. TREASURE, T. and TOSELAND, P. A., Hyperglycaemia due to phenytoin toxicity, *Arch. Dis. Child.*, 46: 563-564, 1971.

1625. TUCHWEBER, B., SZABO, S., KOVACS, K., and GARG, B. D., Hormonal and nonhormonal factors influencing pyrrolizidine alkaloid hepatotoxicity, *Int. Symp. Hepatotoxicity*, 89, 1973.

1626. TURNER, W. J., Dilantin effect on emotionally disturbed children, *Drugs and Cerebral Function*, 99-102, Smith, W. L., Ed., Charles C. Thomas, 1970.   *13*

1627. TYLER, F. H., WEST, C. D., JUBIZ, W., and MEIKLE, A. W., Dilantin and metyrapone: a clinically significant example of enzyme induction, *Trans. Amer. Clin. Climat. Assoc.*, 81: 213-219, 1970.   *81*

1628. TYRER, J. H., EADIE, M. J., and SUTHERLAND, J. M., Investigation of an outbreak of anticonvulsant intoxication, *Proc. Aust. Assoc. Neurol.*, 7: 15-18, 1970.

1629. TYRER, J. H., EADIE, M. J., and HOOPER, W. D., Further observations on an outbreak of diphenylhydantoin intoxication, *Proc. Aust. Assoc. Neurol.*, 8: 37-41, 1971.

1630. UHLENHUTH, E. H., STEPHENS, J. H., DIM, B. H., and COVI, L., Diphenylhydantoin and phenobarbital in the relief of psychoneurotic symptoms: a controlled comparison, *Psychopharmacologia* (Berlin), 27: 67-84, 1972.

1631. UONO, M., Treatment of myotonic dystrophy, *Naika*, 25: 664-668, 1970.

1632. VAISRUB, S., Diphenylhydantoin and insulin-secreting tumors, *JAMA*, 223: 553-554, 1973.

1633. VAISRUB, S., Diphenylhydantoin and early diabetes, *JAMA*, 226: 191, 1973.

1634. VAJDA, F. J. E., PRINEAS, R. J., and LOVELL, R. R. H., Interaction between phenytoin and the benzodiazepines, *Epilepsy Abstracts*, 4: 263, 1971.

1635. VAJDA, F. J. E., PRINEAS, R. J., LOVELL, R. R. H., and SLOMAN, J. G., The possible effect of long-term high plasma levels of phenytoin on mortality after acute myocardial infarction, *Europ. J. Clin. Pharmacol.*, 5: 138-144, 1973.

1636. VAN DER KLEIJN, E., RIJNTJES, N. V. M., GUELEN, P. J. M., and WIJFFELS, C. C. G., Systemic and brain distribution of diphenylhydantoin in the squirrel monkey, *Antiepileptic Drugs*, 124, WOODBURY, D. M., PENRY, J. K., and SCHMIDT, R. P., Eds., Raven Press, New York, 1972.

1637. VAN DER VELDE, C. D., Toxicity of lithium carbonate in elderly patients, *Amer. J. Psychiat.*, 127: 1075-1077, 1971.   *86*

1638. VAN DIJK, L., Pharmacotherapy of cardiac arrhythmias in acute myocardial infarction, *Folia Med. Neerl.*, 14: 225-236, 1971.

1639. VAN METER, J. C., BUCKMASTER, H. S., and SHELLEY, L. L., Concurrent assay of phenobarbital and diphenylhydantoin in plasma by vapor-phase chromatography, *Clin. Chem.*, 16: 135-138, 1970.

1640. VAN REES, H. and NOACH, E. L., The intestinal absorption of diphenylhydantoin from a suspension in rats, *Epilepsy Abstracts*, 7: 197, 1974.

1641. VAN REES, H., DeWOLFF, F. A., NOACH, E. L., The influence of diphenylhydantoin on intestinal glucose absorption in the rat; *European J. Pharmacology*, 28: 310-315, 1974.

1642. VAN REES, H., WOODBURY, D. M. and Noach, E. L., Effects of ouabain and diphenylhydantoin on electrolyte and water shifts during intestinal absorption in the rat, *Arch. Int. Pharmacodyn.*, 182: 437, 1969.   *71*

1643. VAN RIEZEN, H. and DELVER, A., The effect of a number of drugs with different pharmacological properties upon reserpine induced hypothermia in mice, *Arzneimittelforschung.*, 21: 1562-1566, 1971.   *87*

1644. VANASIN, B., BASS, D. D., MENDELOFF, A. I., and SCHUSTER, M. M., Alteration of electrical and motor activity of human and dog rectum by diphenylhydantoin, *Amer. J. Dig. Dis.*, 18: 403-410, 1973.   *72*

1645. VANDER ARK, C. R. and REYNOLDS, E. W. JR., Cellular basis and clinical evaluation of antiarrhythmic therapy, *Med. Clin. N. Amer.*, 53: 1297-1308, 1969.

1646. VAUGHAN WILLIAMS, E. M., The development of new antidysrhythmic drugs, *Schweiz. Med. Wschr.*, 103: 262-271, 1973.

1647. VEDSO, S., RUD, C., and PLACE, J. F., Determination of phenytoin in serum in the presence of barbiturates sulthiame and ethosuximid by thin-layer chromatography, *Scand. J. Clin. Lab. Invest.*, 23: 175-180, 1969.

1648. VEREBEL, K., KUTT, H., SOHN, Y. J., LEVITT, B., and RAINES, A., Uptake and distribution of diphenylthiohydantoin (DPTH), *Europ. J. Pharmacol.*, 10: 106-110, 1970.

1649. VILLAREALE, M., GOULD, L. V., WASSERMAN, R. H., BARR, A., CHIROFF, R. T., and BERGSTROM, W. H., Diphenylhydantoin: effects on calcium metabolism in the chick, *Science*, 183: 671-673, 1974.

1650. VIUKARI, N. M. A. and TAMMISTO, P., Central effects of diphenylhydantoin (Dilantin) in epileptic oligophrenics during phenobarbital-primidone withdrawal, sodium bicarbonate, and ammonium chloride administration, *Behav. Neuropsychiatr.*, 1: 13-16, 1969.

1651. VIUKARI, N. M. A., Diphenylhydantoin as an anticonvulsant: evaluation of treatment in forty mentally subnormal epileptics, *Epilepsy Abstracts*, 3: 150, 1970.

1652. VULLIAMY, D., Unwanted effects of anticonvulsant drugs, *Dev. Med. Child. Neurol.*, 13: 107-109, 1971.

1653. WALKER, W. J., Treatment of heart failure, *JAMA*, 228: 1276-1278, 1974.

1654. WALLACE, J. E., Microdetermination of diphenylhydantoin in biological specimens by ultraviolet spectrophotometry, *Anal. Chem.*, 40: 978-980, 1968.

1655. WALLACE, J. E., Simultaneous spectrophotometric determination of diphenylhydantoin and phenobarbital in biologic specimens, *Clin. Chem.*, 15: 323-330, 1969.

1656. WALLACE, J. E., Spectrophotometric determination of diphenylhydantoin, *J. Forensic Sci. Soc.*, 11: 552-559, 1966.

1657. WALLIS, W. E. and PLUM, F., Continuous fasciculations, myokymia and muscle contraction due to peripheral nerve disease, *Trans. Assoc. Amer. Physicians*, 82: 286-292, 1969.

1658. WALLIS, W. E., VAN POZNAK, A., and PLUM, F., Generalized muscular stiffness, fasciculations, and myokymia of peripheral nerve origin, *Arch. Neurol.*, 22: 430-439, 1970.   *42*

1659. WALSH, G. O., MASLAND, W., and GOLDENSOHN, E. S., Relationship between paroxysmal atrial tachycardia and paroxysmal cerebral discharges, *Bull. Los Angeles Neurol. Soc.*, 37: 28-35, 1972.

1660. WARE, E., The chemistry of the hydantoins, *Chem. Rev.*, 46: 403-470, 1950.

1661. WATANABE, Y., A-V conduction disturbance: its pathophysiology and pharmacology, *Singapore Med. J.*, 14(3): 249, 1973.

1662. WATSON, E. L. and WOODBURY, D. M., Effect of diphenylhydantoin on active sodium transport in frog skin, *J. Pharmacol. Exp. Ther.*, 180: 767-776, 1972.

1663. WATSON, E. L. and WOODBURY, D. M., The effect of diphenylhydantoin and ouabain, alone and in combination, on the electrocardiogram and on cellular electrolytes of guinea-pig heart and skeletal muscle, *Arch. Int. Pharmacodyn.*, 201: 389-399, 1973.   *34*

1664. WATSON, E. L. and WOODBURY, D. M., Effects of diphenylhydantoin on electrolyte transport in various tissues, *Chemical Modulation of Brain Function*, 187-198, SABELLI, H. C., Ed., Raven Press, New York, 1973.   *64*

1665. WATSON, J. D. and SPELLACY, W. N., Neonatal effects of maternal treatment with the anticonvulsant drug diphenylhydantoin, *Obstet. Gynec.*, 37: 881-885, 1971.

1666. WATSON, M., GABICA, J., and BENSON, W. W., Serum organochlorine pesticides in mentally retarded patients on differing drug regimens, *Clin. Pharmacol. Ther.*, 13: 186-192, 1972.   *85*

1667. WATSON, P., Brainwave to save life, *London Times*, 1973.

REFERENCES

1668. WAX, S. D., WEBB, W. R., and ECKER, R. R., Myocardium stabilization by diphenylhydantoin, *Surg. Forum*, 20: 164-166, 1969. *33*

1669. WEBER-EGGENBERGER, S. and KAUFMANN, G., Studies on absorption, elimination and antiarrhythmic serum concentrations of diphenylhydantoin (antisacer) in digitalized heart patients, *Z. Kreislaufforsch.*, 60: 420-432, 1971.

1670. WECKMAN, N. and LEHTOVAARA, R., Serum and cerebrospinal fluid folate values in epileptics on anticonvulsant treatment, *Scand. J. Clin. Lab. Invest.*, Supp. 101, 120-121, 1968.

1671. WECKMAN, N. and LEHTOVAARA, R., Folic acid and anticonvulsants, *Lancet*, 1: 207-208, 1969.

1672. WEINREICH, D. and CLARK, L. D., Anticonvulsant drugs and self-stimulation rates in rats, *Arch. Int. Pharmacodyn.*, 185: 269-273, 1970.

1673. WEISSE, A. B., MOSCHOS, C. B., PASSANNANTE, A. J., and REGAN, T. J., Comparative effectiveness of procaine amide, lidocaine, and diphenylhydantoin in treating ventricular arrhythmias during acute myocardial infarction, *Circulation*, 38: VI205, 1968.

1674. WEISS, C. F., YAFFE, S. J., CANN, H. M., GOLD, A. P., KENNY, F. M., RILEY, H. D., SCHAFER, I., STERN, L., and SHIRKEY, H. C., An evaluation of the pharmacologic approaches to learning impediments, *Pediatrics*, 46: 142-144, 1970.

1675. WEISSE, A. B., MOSCHOS, C. B., PASSANNANTE, A. J., KHAN, M. I., and REGAN, T. J., Relative effectiveness of three anti-arrhythmic agents in the treatment of ventricular arrhythmias in experimental acute myocardial ischemia, *Amer. Heart J.*, 81: 503-510, 1971.

1676. WELCH, L. K., APPENZELLER, O., and BICKNELL, J. M., Peripheral neuropathy with myokymia, sustained muscular contraction, and continuous motor unit activity, *Neurology*, 22: 161-169, 1972. *42*

1677. WEPSIC, J. G., Tic douloureux: etiology, refined treatment, *New Eng. J. Med.*, 288: 680-681, 1973.

1678. WERK, E. E., CHOI, Y., SHOLITON, L., OLINGER, C., and HAQUE, N., Interference in the effect of dexamethasone by diphenylhydantoin, *New Eng. J. Med.*, 281: 32-34, 1969.

1679. WERK, E. E., THRASHER, K., SHOLITON, L. J., OLINGER, C., and CHOI, Y., Cortisol production in epileptic patients treated with diphenylhydantoin, *Clin. Pharmacol. Ther.*, 12: 698-703, 1971. *80*

1680. WESSELING, H. and THURKOW, I., Effect of sulphonylureas (tolazamide, tolbutamide and chlorpropamide) on the metabolism of diphenylhydantoin in the rat, *Biochem. Pharmacol.*, 22: 3033-3040, 1973.

1681. WESTMORELAND, B. and BASS, N. H., Chronic diphenylhydantoin intoxication in the albino rat during pregnancy, *Neurology*, 20: 411, 1970.

1682. WHELTON, A., SNYDER, D. S., and WALKER, W. G., Acute toxic drug ingestions at the Johns Hopkins Hospital 1963 through 1970, *Johns Hopkins Med. J.*, 132: 157-167, 1973.

1683. WHITE, C. W., Jr., MEGIRIAN, R., and SWISS, E. D., The effects of diphenylhydantoin sodium, glucose and β-diethylaminoethyl diphenylpropylacetate hydrochloride on cyclopropane-epinephrine arrhythmias in the dog, *Circ. Res.*, 3: 290-292, 1955.

1684. WILDER, B. J., BUCHANAN, R. A., and SERRANO, E. E., Correlation of acute diphenylhydantoin intoxication with plasma levels and metabolite excretion, *Neurology*, 23: 1329-1332, 1973.

1685. WILDER, B. J., SERRANO, E. E. and RAMSAY, R. E., Plasma diphenylhydantoin levels after loading and maintenance doses, *Clin. Pharmacol. Ther.*, 14: 797-801, 1973.

1686. WILDER, B. J., STREIFF, R. R., and HAMMER, R. H., Diphenylhydantoin, absorption, distribution, and excretion: clinical studies, *Antiepileptic Drugs*, 137-148, WOODBURY, D. M., PENRY, J. K., and SCHMIDT, R. P., Eds., Raven Press, New York, 1972.

1687. WILENSKY, A. J. and LOWDEN, J. A., Interaction of diphenylhydantoin 4^{14}C with subcellular fractions of rat brain, *Epilepsy Abstracts*, 5: 194, 1972. *93*

1688. WILENSKY, A. J. and LOWDEN, J. A., The inhibitory effect of diphenylhydantoin on microsomal ATPases, *Life Sci.*, 11: 319-327, 1972.

1689. WILENSKY, A. J. and LOWDEN, J. A., Inadequate serum levels after intramuscular administration of diphenylhydantoin, *Neurology*, 23: 318-324, 1973.

1690. WILKINSON, H. A., Epileptic pain—an uncommon manifestation with localizing value, *Neurology*, 23: 518-520, 1973.

1691. WILSON, J. T. and WILKINSON, G. R., Delivery of anticonvulsant drug therapy in epileptic patients assessed by plasma level analyses, *Neurology*, 24: 614-623, 1974.

1692. WINTER, B., Bilateral carotid body resection for asthma and emphysema, *Int. Surg.*, 57: 458-466, 1972.   *49*

1693. WOLFF, J., STANDAERT, M. E., and RALL, J. E., Thyroxine displacement from serum proteins and depression of serum protein-bound iodine by certain drugs, *J. Clin. Invest.*, 40: 1373-1377, 1961.

1694. WOOD, R. A., Sinoatrial arrest: an interaction between phenytoin and lignocaine, *Brit. Med. J.*, 1: 645, 1971.

1695. WOODBURY, D. M. and KEMP, J. W., Some possible mechanisms of action of anti-epileptic drugs, *Pharmakopsychiatr.*, 3: 201-226, 1970.

1696. WOODBURY, D. M. and KEMP, J. W., Pharmacology and mechanisms of action of diphenylhydantoin,   *64* *Psychiat. Neurol. Neurochir.*, 74: 91-115, 1971.

1697. WOODBURY, D. M. and SWINYARD, E. A., Diphenylhydantoin, absorption, distribution, and excretion, *Antiepileptic Drugs*, 113-123, WOODBURY, D. M., PENRY, J. K., and SCHMIDT, R. P., Eds., Raven Press, New York, 1972.

1698. WOODBURY, D. M., KOCH, A., and VERNADAKIS, A., Relation between excitability and metabolism in brain as elucidated by anticonvulsant drugs, *Neurology*, 8: 113-116, 1958.

1699. WOODBURY, D. M., Mechanisms of action of anticonvulsants, *Epilepsy Abstracts*, 3: 248, 1970.

1700. WOODBURY, D. M., PENRY, J. K. and SCHMIDT, R. P., Eds., *Antiepileptic Drugs*, Raven Press, New York,   *53* 1972.

1701. YALAZ, K. and BAYTOK, V., Mirror movement, *Turk. J. Pediat.*, 12: 85-88, 1970.   *47*

1702. YANAGIHARA, T. and HAMBERGER, A., Effect of diphenylhydantoin on protein metabolism in the central nervous system—study of subcellular fractions, *Exp. Neurol*, 31: 87-99, 1971.

1703. YANAGIHARA, T. and HAMBERGER, A., Effect of diphenylhydantoin on protein metabolism in neuron and neuroglial fractions of central nervous tissue, *Exp. Neurol*, 32: 152-162, 1971.

1704. YANAGIHARA, T., Distribution of diphenylhydantoin in the neuronal and glial fractions, *Antiepileptic*   *93* *Drugs*, 125-126, WOODBURY, D. M., PENRY, J. K., and SCHMIDT, R. P., Eds., Raven Press, New York, 1972.

1705. YANG, C. P., Persistent ventricular tachycardia. The use of diphenylhydantoin, *J. Kansas Med. Soc.*, 74:   *27* 418-421, 1973.

1706. YARYURA-TOBIAS, J. A. and NEZIROGLU, F., Violent behaviour, brain dysrhythmia and glucose dysfunction: a new syndrome, *Amer. J. Psychiat.*, 130: 825, 1973.

1707. YASKY, J., MORETTI, O., CAROSELLA, C., Phenytoin treatment of cardiac arrhythmias induced by digitalis,   *86* *Revista Argentina de Cardiologia*, 41: 53-61, 1973.

1708. YOSHIDA, T. and ARAKAWA, T., Serum histidine clearance in children with diphenylhydantoin administration, *Tohoku J. Exp. Med.*, 112: 257-259, 1974.

1709. YOSHIMASU, F., KURLAND, L. T., and ELVEBACK, L. R., Tic douloureux in Rochester, Minnesota, 1945-1969, *Neurology*, 22: 952-956, 1972.

1710. ZANINI, S. and ROSSI, R., Ventricular parasystole: effective treatment with diphenylhydantoin, *G. Ital. Cardiol.*, 2: 575-578, 1972.

1711. ZEFT, H. J., REMBERT, J. C., CURRY, C. L., and GREENFIELD, J. C., Effects of diphenylhydantoin on   *32* coronary and systemic haemodynamics in awake dogs, *Cardiovasc. Res.*, 7: 331-335, 1973.

1712. ZEFT, H. J., WHALEN, R. E., MORRIS, J. J., JR., RUMMO, N. J., and McINTOCH, H. D., Prophylaxis versus treatment of acetylstrophanthidin intoxication, *Amer. Heart J.*, 77: 237-245, 1969.